An Introduction to Growing and Using Culinary and Medicinal Herbs

THE *Beauty of Herbs*

JESSICA DORFSMITH

The Beauty of Herbs
An Introduction to Growing and Using Culinary and Medicinal Herbs
Written by Jessica Dorfsmith

All artwork, text, and poetry marked "J.L.D." by Jessica Dorfsmith, unless otherwise stated. All Scripture quotations from King James Version.

Disclaimer: *This book is not a medical reference. The author and publishers cannot be held responsible for any harmful reactions to the suggestions, recommendations, hints, recipes, tips, or anything contained herein. The author of this book does not profess to be an expert or professional. This book is not intended to take the place of professional medical advice from your doctor or qualified persons. Always consult your physician with medical questions and research carefully before using herbs in any form.*

ISBN: 978-1-933753-32-4

Book design by Rosetta Mullet
Printed by Carlisle Printing of Walnut Creek

Carlisle Press
WALNUT CREEK

2673 Township Road 421
Sugarcreek, Ohio 44681
phone | 800.852.4482

Dedication

I owe the idea for this book to my mother. Without her suggestions and encouragement, it would have remained an unrealized dream. Thank you, Mom—it is to you that I dedicate this book.

Special thanks to my sister Susannah for carefully checking over the rough draft and cheering me on each step of the way.

Contents

Living Proof

For the cattle, there's grass
In the wide-spreading field;
Where they graze, picturesque and at ease.
And here in the garden,
As I bend to my work,
Now I pause for a bit on my knees;
My gaze is taking in
The bright herbs as they grow,
And the food that comes forth from the ground.
And I smile, for I know
It's the blessing of God
Making all these good things to abound.
So while here on my knees,
Midst my toil and God's gifts,
My whole heart is quick-lifted in prayer,
Of glad thanks to the Lord
Who has given to me
Living proof of His hand everywhere.
–J.L.D.

Introduction to Herbs

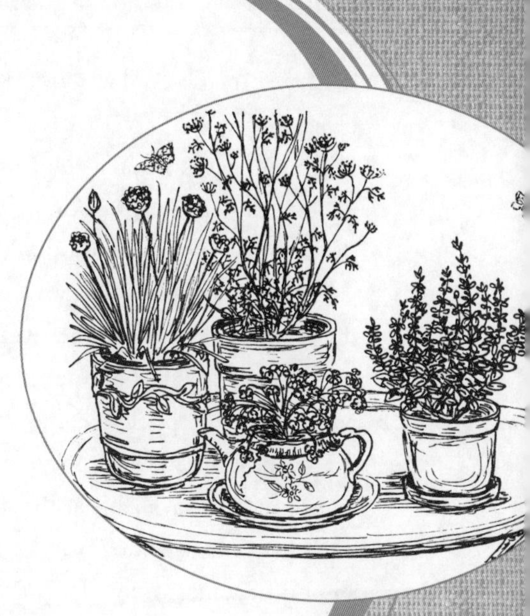

He causeth the grass to grow for the cattle, and herb for the service of man: that he may bring forth food out of the earth (Psalm 104:14).

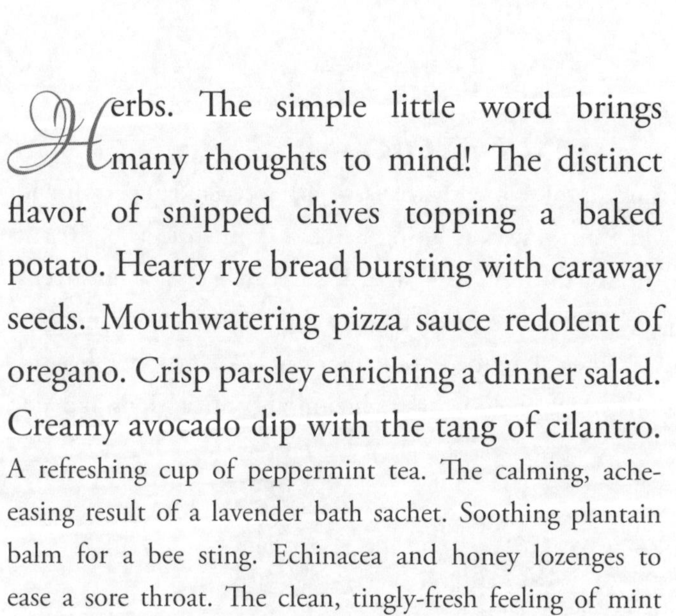

Herbs. The simple little word brings many thoughts to mind! The distinct flavor of snipped chives topping a baked potato. Hearty rye bread bursting with caraway seeds. Mouthwatering pizza sauce redolent of oregano. Crisp parsley enriching a dinner salad. Creamy avocado dip with the tang of cilantro. A refreshing cup of peppermint tea. The calming, ache-easing result of a lavender bath sachet. Soothing plantain balm for a bee sting. Echinacea and honey lozenges to ease a sore throat. The clean, tingly-fresh feeling of mint toothpaste. And the list goes on—and on!

Sometimes unrecognized, herbs are in the ingredient list of many products we use daily and they frequently find their way into our cooking and home remedies. Few of us can look over the past week and not find at least one or two herbs in our consumption, topical use, oral care, medicinal, or home care use. And why not? Herbs offer a wide spectrum of naturally healthful benefits.

To me, herbs are an awe-inspiring proof of our Creator's all-wise provision for us. "He causeth the grass to grow for the cattle, and herb for the service of man: that he may bring forth food out of the earth" (Psalm 104:14).

The implication of this verse is that gardening requires two things to succeed: the blessing of God and the sweat of the brow. In my experience, this has proven true! Gardening in the Rocky Mountains of southwest Colorado (with our short growing season, poor soil, and the unpredictable weather) isn't effortless—to put it mildly. Maybe you can relate! Sometimes friends ask me, "Why do you work so hard? Herbs are available at the health or grocery store. Can't you just buy those?" The answer is, I sometimes do! But since few enjoyments beat that of working among fragrant, lovely plants that are also useful, delicious, and healthy, I don't mind the effort!

MY STORY

I am not an expert or a professional herbalist—just an everyday person who intensely enjoys studying, growing, and using herbs. My interest in herbs and natural health began nearly thirteen years ago. I was barely out of my teens, suffering from a sluggish colon due to spinal damage and miserable with inflamed complexion problems. I knew I needed something to help me—but what? I shrank from medications which included a frightening list of cautions and side

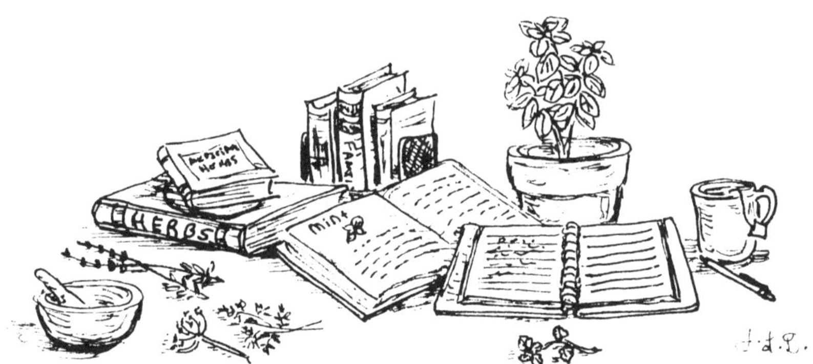

effects, but desperation drove me to try what several doctors suggested. To my dismay, the medications offered poor results along with health hazards. What was I to do?

At that time my mother (who has always had an interest in herbs) purchased a book on medicinal herbs. It opened a whole new way of life! Mom had always kept an aloe vera plant in the kitchen for treating burns, plus she often used herbs in cooking, but using herbs as medicine was still untried territory for us.

Together we began researching natural remedies for my colon health. (I had discovered, shortly before this, that good old aloe vera was the answer to my complexion problems, but more on that later!) The result was a wonderful answer to prayer. God supplied relief for my needs in a natural, safe, and effective manner. And that was the beginning of my interest and work with herbs.

Although medicinal herbs first caught my attention, culinary herbs soon joined the ranks. And I have since discovered that there is even more enjoyment to herbs than I at first imagined. What can beat the fun of growing herbs for their beauty, versatility, and usefulness? There's a particular pleasure in being out-of-doors in God's creation, my hands in the warm soil and the fragrant, lovely plants thriving around me! Relishing the citrusy, tangy, spicy, sweet, or savory taste in foods and beverages; carefully making use of medicinal qualities; investigating essential oils; and simply introducing the use of herbs into the various aspects of daily life is an enjoyment I wouldn't want to be without.

If you have never ventured to grow or use herbs, I hope these pages will encourage you to begin. If you are an experienced herbalist, may you find pleasant enjoyment walking among tried-and-true "old friends."

> *All the flowers of tomorrow are in the seeds of today.*
> *–Unknown*

THREE RULES FOR USING HERBS

Carefully avoid New Age or witchcraft influences sometimes associated with herbs. Accept herbs for what they are: a gift from God for the benefit of man, to be properly used and never abused.

Use herbs wisely. Don't blindly rush in, trying this herb or that. Some herbs are not for ingestion; some should never be given to children; some pose risks for those with heart disease, high blood pressure, etc.; some are not to be used by pregnant women. Be wise—do your research!

Don't be intimidated. Growing, using, preserving, and learning about herbs may take time, but you'll find it well spent!

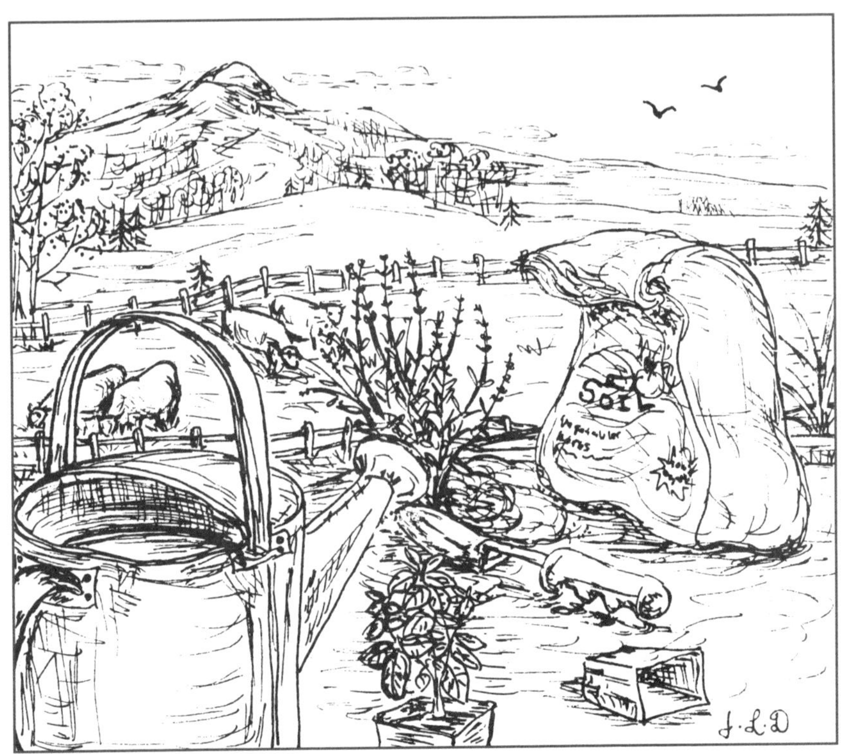

The Herb Garden

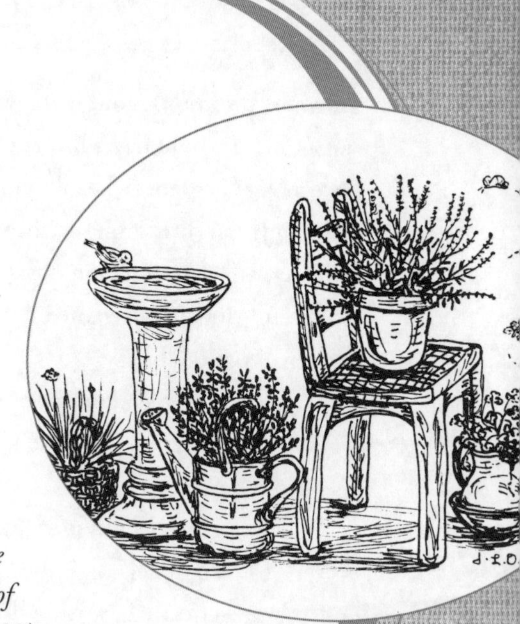

The LORD ...said, ...[I have] divided a watercourse for the overflowing of waters, ...a way for the lightning of thunder; To cause it to rain on the earth, ...to cause the bud of the tender herb to spring forth (Job 38:1-27).

I thoroughly enjoy the versatility of herb gardening! It can be as simple or complex as you choose. If you are new to growing herbs, perhaps you're wondering just where to start. Or maybe you already have a lovely garden, but are eager to use your creativity and branch out! Whatever the case, there are a myriad of ideas. In this chapter we'll briefly cover a few.

PART ONE: CONTAINER GARDENING

Usually container gardening is suggested for those who have small yards, tight schedules, or poor growing conditions. And it *is* a wonderful solution for such problems! But at the same time, I would never limit container gardening to those instances. Even if you have a huge garden, rich soil, and plenty of time, a charming pot of lime basil, an old bundt pan brimming with brilliant green curled parsley, a barrel of fragrant lavender, another of lemongrass, and a long, low container of peppermint make a wonderful, low maintenance retreat when grouped around a comfortable bench and small patio table.

We like to keep containers of most-used culinary herbs on our back deck (just steps from the kitchen!) where it is convenient to harvest small amounts of what we need when we need it.

Certain herbs are also useful in warding off mosquitoes, flies, and other pesky visitors to your deck or patio. Portable containers of tansy, fennel, lavender, and rue are effective. Scatter brimming pots all around to improve your next summertime outdoor event!

Container herb gardening is a good outlet for your creativity. An old stockpot, chipped pitcher, leaky washtub, or any number of containers work well—and look lovely when graced with herbs! Keep in mind that herbs you expect to use for topical, medicinal, or culinary purposes should be grown in food-safe containers.

When choosing herbs for containers, find what type of soil and conditions each herb thrives in, then plant accordingly. Most potted herbs find compacted soil suffocating and keel over in a soggy environment. Purchasing a quality potting mix is a good start, but I suggest adding perlite, vermiculite, and composted organic matter to the mix. This keeps the soil light and well drained. And remember, containers need adequate drainage holes. If this isn't possible, add a layer of small pebbles to the bottom of the container.

Each potted herb has individual watering needs—it helps to do your research! Some like their foliage misted, some require the soil to completely dry between watering, and so forth. A good rule of thumb for the average potted herb, though, is to keep the soil evenly moist—not too wet, but not allowing it to completely dry out. In extremely dry climates, adding a layer of mulch around your potted herbs is a good idea. This helps retain moisture.

Don't think that just because your herbs aren't out there in a traditional herb garden, they won't need fertilizer! It's helpful to add an all-purpose fertilizer several times throughout the growing season. I usually apply a water-soluble formula that feeds both the roots and foliage.

Treat potted perennials as you would those in the garden—unless they can also act as evergreens and you plan on moving them into your greenhouse for the winter. Cut back and mulch those staying out-of-doors, and remember to uncover and water in the spring!

Container herbs indoors? Yes, it has been done—and with success. However, don't expect your indoor herbs to thrive as they do out-of-doors or in a greenhouse environment. The fullness of flavor is also sacrificed (aloe vera is the exception), and the life span rather uncertain.

Despite these facts, I have a lovely lemon thyme plant beautifying a hanging basket by the window near my desk, and a perky lime basil in a pot on the windowsill next to my aloe vera. They add a bright spot and look cheery—even when it's snowy outside!

Some good choices for indoor herbs are aloe vera, thyme, basil, oregano, and parsley. Contrary to those lovely pictures you may see of chive plants in a kitchen windowsill, I do not recommend it. Chives need cool outdoor weather to produce their delicious flavor.

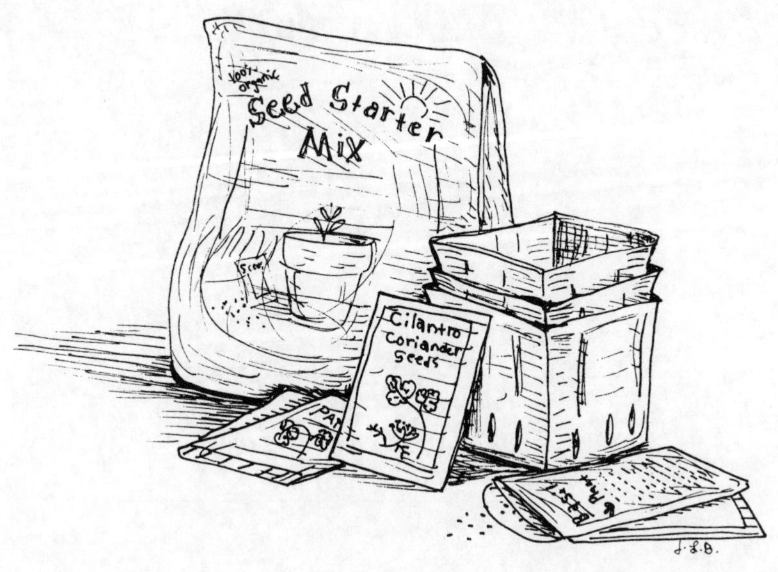

Use the same type of potting mix you use for outdoor potted herbs, unless they have special soil requirements (aloe vera, for example, needs a cacti/succulent potting mix). You might need to water more frequently indoors, but don't let the soil get soggy, and be absolutely sure to keep the pots in a sunny location. In the spring, add an all-purpose fertilizer.

TOP TEN CHOICES FOR CONTAINER GARDENING

Bush Basil	Chives
Lavender	Lemongrass
Mint	Oregano
Parsley	Sage
Savory	Thyme

IMPRESSIVE POTTED HERBS

Bay	Lavender
Lemongrass	Myrtle
Rosemary	Juniper

Gardens are not made by singing,
"Oh, how beautiful," and sitting in the shade.
–Rudyard Kipling

PART TWO: ROCK GARDENS AND WILD GARDENS

Many herbs grow in the wild, which is a good indication of their hardy constitution! And guess what—this feature opens a vast amount of gardening design opportunities. What can be prettier than a rustic stone wall brimming with low-maintenance creeping thyme, yarrow, lavender, peppermint, and prostrate rosemary? Or how about a pile of big rocks as a centerpiece, with hardy herbs growing amongst them? Another unique idea is to cover a hillside with cascading herbs that thrive in poor soil and rocky conditions. And then there are such delightful possibilities for filling a sunny, open area with herbs whose natural habitat is in the wild!

A rock garden will need little attention—but yes, it *will* need a little! Adding organic matter to the soil is a must, and be sure to keep your plants watered if rain isn't plentiful. Choose tough, easy-to-grow herbs that require well-drained rocky or sandy soil and have trailing habits. Herbs like lavender and yarrow are good too, because their bushy beauty naturally (and gracefully!) leans over rock walls,

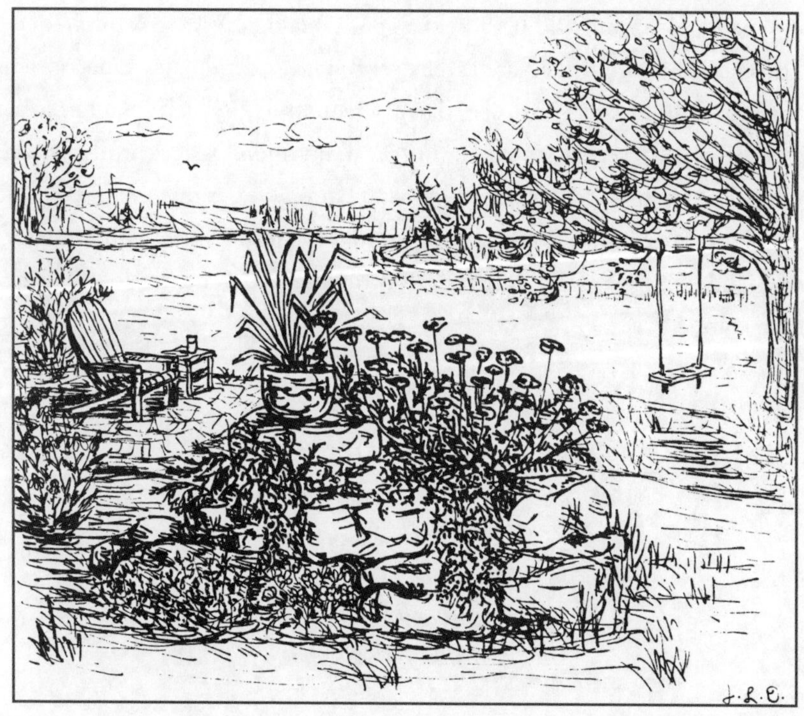

planters, piles of rock, and rocky outcroppings. You may want to add bright little flowering herbs (such as California poppies, violets, and nasturtiums) for a burst of cheery color.

A plain, uninteresting hillside can be turned into a breathtakingly, beautiful sight with a bit of effort and some hardy herbs! If the hillside is steep, you will need to design terraces that step down, keeping the soil from erosion (which will leave your herbs to starve and thirst to death!).

If the slope is shallow and sprawling, however, you can usually get rugged herbs to thrive. Yes, adding organic matter to the soil is a must, and once the plants are established, don't forget to water them! Other than that, your job will simply be to exclaim, "How pretty!" whenever you happen to glance at your herb-cascading hillside!

All of the herbs that do well in a rock garden should thrive on your hillside. Look especially for the trailing type, and for herbs that make good ground cover.

To create a wild herb field, clear an open area that gets full sun. Till in organic matter. Treat it much as you would a wildflower field. In the fall or early spring, scatter seeds, lightly cover, and in the spring keep moist until they germinate. If rain is sparse, give your wild herb field a good soaking every week or two.

The choices for your field are extensive! Borage, calendula, echinacea, fennel, sunflower, St.-John's-wort, oxeye daisy, chamomile, alfalfa, plantain, black-eyed Susan, rue, feverfew, mullein, and so many more! Check into each herb's individual needs and provide accordingly. Or simply experiment and see if they'll thrive when treated as wild vegetation. In my experience, most will! Many of the herbs mentioned self-seed effortlessly too, making your field a lovely sight for years to come.

Grandmother's garden had old-fashioned flowers—
Hollyhocks, roses, and rue.
And Grandmother dear, in her quaint little gown,
Was an old-fashioned, sweet flower too!
–Miriam Ott Munson

Out in the Fields with God

The little cares that fretted me, I lost them yesterday,
Among the fields, above the sea, among the winds at play;
Among the lowing of the herds, the rustling of the trees;
Among the singing of the birds, the humming of the bees.
The foolish fears of what may happen, I cast them all away,
Among the clover-scented grass, among the new-mown hay;
Among the rustling of the corn, where drowsy poppies nod,
Where ill thoughts die and good are born—
Out in the fields with God.
–Elizabeth Barrett Browning

PART THREE: RAISED BEDS, BORDERS, AND WALKWAYS

These are actually my favorite type of herb gardens. The design possibilities are nearly limitless, and you can fit them almost anywhere!

Raised beds are an excellent choice if your soil is poor—but that isn't the only reason for them! They make it a lot easier on your back when working among the herbs, plus you won't pack down the soil by walking on it to weed and harvest. Also, if you want to add dimension to your yard, this is a good way to do it.

You can make raised beds out of so many different materials. Make tidy redwood boxes, rustic planters of stacked rocks, wooden beams, logs, and more! Or use those convenient landscaping blocks you'll find at your local hardware or garden supply.

For years folks have used railroad ties or treated wood for raised beds. That's fine for ornamental flowers, but *never* for herbs or vegetables! The toxins in the railroad ties and treated wood will end up leeching into the soil and contaminating your plants. This poses serious risks, blotting out a main reason for growing your own herbs and vegetables—your health!

When planning where to put raised beds, it's helpful to draw a simple sketch before you get to work. Then mark the dimensions of the area at the site and till the soil. Build your raised beds around the tilled area. Bring in topsoil and add lots of organic matter to fill the beds ¾ full. Then choose the herbs you want and plant accordingly! Oh yes, and raised beds are excellent if you want to do a theme garden, but more on that later!

Herb borders are especially nice in small yards. Many herbs grow in tidy bushes or easy-to-trim hedges, and they are ideal for this purpose. Be sure to plant tall herbs at the back and smaller herbs towards the front.

Among the dozens of choices for borders are lavender, rosemary, sage, catnip, comfrey, chives (or any of the *Allium* genus), all mints, horehound, tarragon, winter savory, myrtle, southernwood, anise hyssop, garden thyme, bay, and chamomile.

Herbs are a lovely way to edge your lawn. This ties in with raised beds, since that's probably the way you will want to do it. A raised bed prevents grass from invading the herbs, and helps keep out harmful chemicals used in lawns.

Walkways are absolutely picturesque when you incorporate herbs! Use your imagination. There are so many possibilities. And this ties in with borders, since

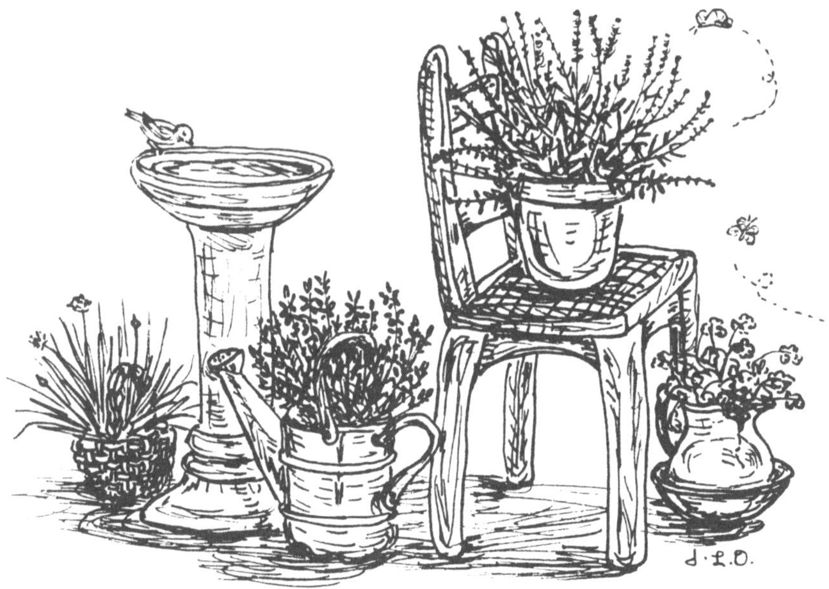

walkways are best with a border of plants on either side.

Why not set a comfy bench in a corner of your yard, perhaps beside that giant lilac? Next, lay out two garden hoses—these will be the guide for shaping your walkway! Gracefully curve the hoses into the form you want. Level dirt where needed. Add a layer of sand or pea gravel if you want to, then lay the path with brick, stone, pavers, stepping stones, or whatever you choose. Make sure you leave space to plant creeping thyme and mint among them. (Okay, you can put away the garden hoses now!) Along the outside edge of your path, till up the soil and add organic matter. Plant chamomile, feverfew, lavender, catnip, all types of mint, lemon balm, and any fragrant herbs you choose. These will give off a wonderfully pleasant aroma when brushed against (or stepped on!) while walking along the path. Now, at the end of the path, group various-sized pots filled with lemongrass, rosemary, etc. around your bench. Bring out a frosty pitcher of lemonade (flavored with a bit of peppermint, of course!), a tall glass of ice, and a good book. Settle down on the bench and relax!

PART FOUR: THE FORMAL HERB GARDEN

Formal herb gardens are carefully planned and precisely ordered arrangements. They usually follow a specific pattern and are kept neatly trimmed to retain their shape. A centerpiece or focal point—whether it be a sundial, large potted herb (such as bay), gazebo, bench, etc.—is usually prominent.

The visual charm of orderly formal herb gardens make them as well-loved today as they have been for centuries. They are painstakingly spaced, shaped, and divided. So, yes, this type of garden is far more difficult to lay out, plant, establish, and maintain! Two main keys are to lay them out in a way which allows the plants to get as much sun as possible, and to make each section accessible without treading on the plants!

Some simple and lovely formal designs are as follows:

The pie shape, or wagon wheel shape, in which walkways go between each wedge, and a centerpiece is placed in the middle. The wedges may each be planted alike, or each contain a different theme. Usually they are edged with well-trimmed shrubby herbs.

The checkerboard garden— You may use garden stones of any size, but let's say 12" squares as an example. They are spaced to make a checkerboard with 12" squares of soil. In the soil (enriched as you would any garden), plant one type of herb per square. This design is also excellent for themes.

The ladder garden is made in the shape of a tall ladder lying down. Herbs are planted between each "rung." The "rungs" and "ladder" parts can be made with wood, stones, etc., and yes, even with the real thing! This type of arrangement is especially pretty when made from herbs that form hedges and can be trimmed to the ladder shape. Rosemary, winter savory, and garden thyme are a few good choices for the "ladder" part. Each "rung" can contain different herbs, like oregano, lavender, echinacea, lemon balm, etc. The ladder design is perfect for putting on either side of a straight, formal walkway, perhaps leading to a gazebo.

Go ahead and design your own formal herb garden! There are so many fun ideas. Why not try a favorite quilt block design, such as the Ohio Star? Instead of different fabrics, you'll incorporate different shades of herbs. Add narrow walkways between the blocks, making a large "quilt." Put a trellis at one side with climbing roses on it for your "headboard." Add a bench at the foot. Now that's charming!

Or how about making a garden in the shape of a giant sunflower, with a graceful "stem" and a couple of "leaves"? In the center, plant some large chocolate mint bushes. Have the "petals" filled with yellow or creamy flowering herbs. Plant curled parsley and well-trimmed chives in the "stem" and "leaf" areas. How pretty!

Or have you ever thought of having a graceful cascade of herbs, carefully shaped like a winding river, spilling down a gentle incline? You could have rows of different flowering herbs growing in ribbons down the "river," making a rainbow of color.

As I said, there are so many fun ideas!

PART FIVE: THEME GARDENS

Herbs planted in separate small gardens, each with its own theme, is gardening at its best! It's also good for the beginning herb gardener, preventing confusion between culinary and medicinal herbs. Raised beds are my choice for theme herb gardens, but you may easily incorporate themes into your formal herb gardens as well.

The following ideas are simply that: ideas! Use them as a springboard to get your imagination running. Choose herbs that do best in your climate, suit your family's medicinal needs, and please your eyes and taste buds.

Tea-Time Garden— You need a relaxing cup of steaming hot tea. Imagine yourself stepping outside and strolling to a pretty bed of herbs, each one healthful and delicious in tea. Harvest your choice, put some water on to boil, and get out your teapot!

Mint—any variety *(the more the better!)*	Chamomile
Lemon balm	Catnip
Lemon thyme	Fennel
Lime and lemon basil	Bergamot *(also called bee balm)*

Culinary Herb Garden— These herbs are top choices for the kitchen and grow well in containers. Arrange some brimming pots on your patio!

Chives	Savory
Basil	Sage
Oregano	Parsley
Cilantro/coriander	Thyme

> *As for marigolds, poppies, hollyhocks, and valorous sunflowers, we shall never have a garden without them, both for their own sake and for the sake of old-fashioned folks who used to love them.*
> *–Henry Ward Beecher*

Immune-Builder Garden— These herbs are excellent for treating the common cold and flu, while building your immune system and overall health!

Echinacea	Horehound
Chamomile	Horseradish
Peppermint	Lemon balm
Mullein	Rosemary

Edible Flower Herb Garden— Flowers are usually so pretty that we might exclaim, "Those look good enough to eat!" And guess what—many herb flowers are! A pretty design for this theme is having a well-trimmed rosebush as the center, with flagstones around it and petal shapes coming from the middle.

Roses	Violets
Bergamot	Chives
Chamomile	Rosemary
Chicory	Red clover
Chrysanthemum	Calendula
California poppy	

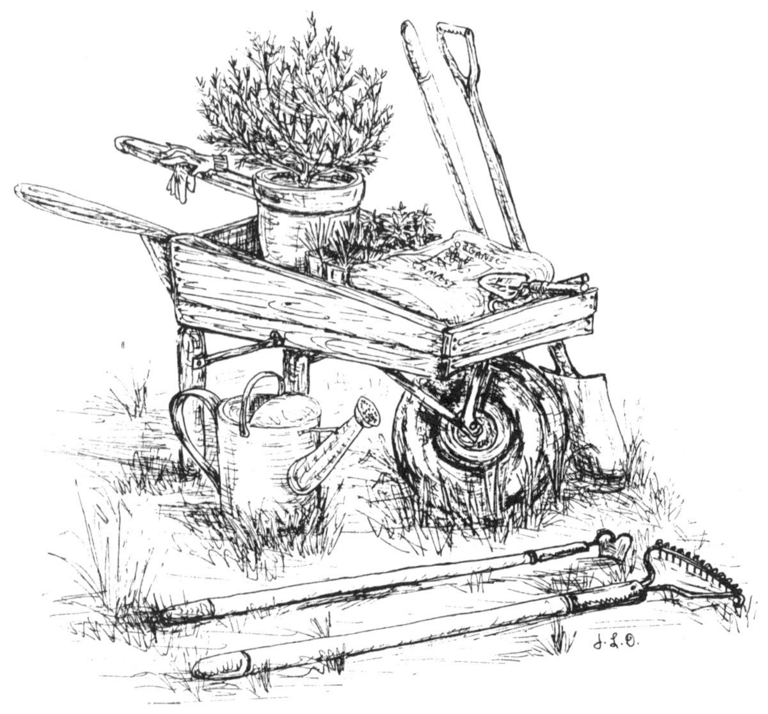

Butterfly and Bee Herb Garden— I love this one! It's fragrant, lovely, and always buzzing with activity! You might want to place this garden near your fruit trees. Remember to situate it where there is full sun! Oh, and it's a good idea to scatter plantain (whose leaves are soothing to stings) among the other herbs, just in case you happen to get a bee sting while admiring your garden!

Borage	Horehound
Echinacea	Savory
Oregano	Mint
Thyme	Marjoram
Rosemary	Anise hyssop
Catnip	Red clover
Bergamot	Sage

There are so many possibilities for arranging herb gardens. It may take some experimenting to find what's best for your family's needs, but there are dozens of gardening books brimming with advice. Why not check out a few from your local library, get some paper and a pencil, and start planning your own herb garden today?!

GROWING TIPS

Fish fertilizer (available through Berlin Seeds, see page 223) works wonders with herbs. It's great for foliage feeding, resulting in lush, healthy growth. It also promotes seed germination, and improves the soil too!

Water-soluble all-purpose formulas (such as Miracle-Gro™) are safe and effective.

Homemade Bug Spray

A good spray, attacking soft-bodied pests like aphids, mealy bugs, and spider mites.

1 gallon warm water

1 teaspoon liquid dish soap

1 teaspoon cooking oil

Mix well. Add to a spray bottle and spray daily for three days.

For fighting mildew, fungus, and diseases, simply add 2 tablespoons of baking soda to the mix above.

My Herb Garden

There's lavender with stately form,
And wholesome, sweet perfume;
A patch of silv'ry rosemary,
Light blue when it's in bloom.
Low-growing bed of peppermint,
Delightful as to smell;
Then delicate the foliage of
Savory sweet basil.

A bushy clump of lemongrass,
Like citrus in its scent;
And the cilantro's foliage like
A frost with bright green tint.
The mullein's standing strong and tall,
The garden at its feet:
And thyme is creeping round the stones,
Making the path complete.
–J.L.D.

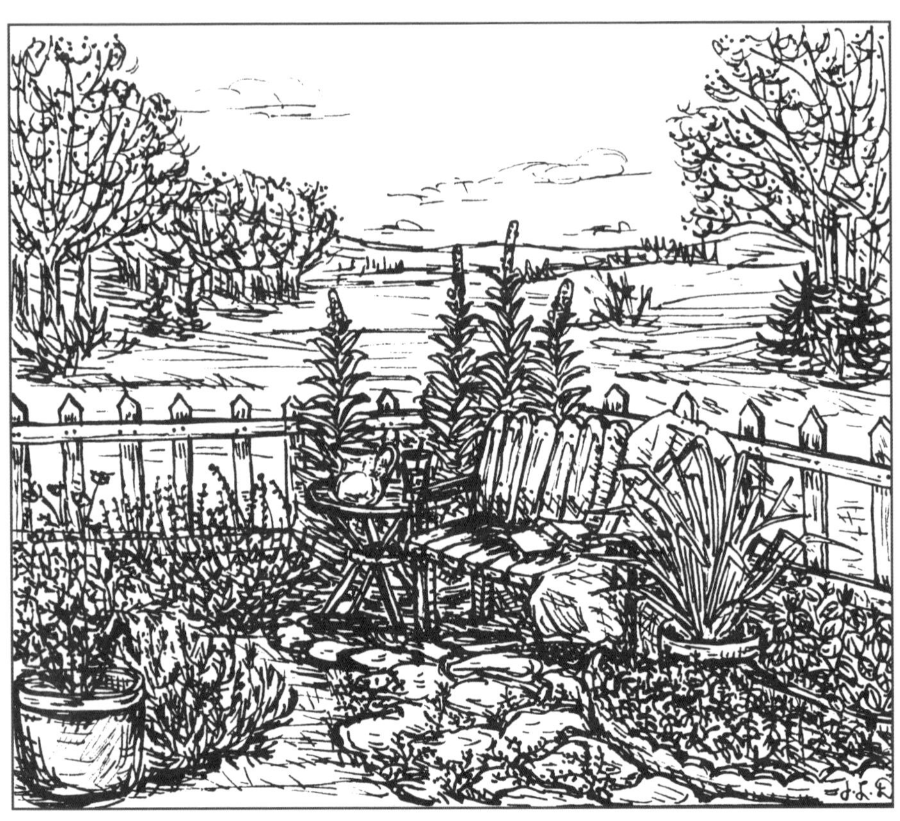

Top Fifteen Culinary Herbs

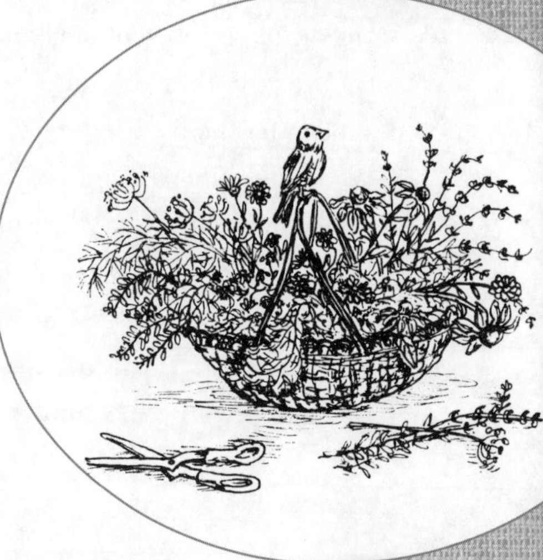

I will praise thee, O LORD, with my whole heart; I will shew forth all thy marvelous works (Psalm 9:1).

"Out of so many useful herbs, how can I trim each category down to fifteen favorites?" Such was the dilemma I faced in the early planning stages of this book! But with effort and discipline I managed to narrow it down to what I believe to be a well-rounded, worthwhile variety.

"Culinary" is the title given to herbs primarily used in the kitchen. Fresh or dried, they lend a citrusy, tangy, spicy, sweet, savory, or hot flavor to many dishes we make every day. What would life be like without culinary herbs? Imagine how bland spaghetti sauce, poultry stuffing, cheese spreads, rye bread, pickles, and so many other dishes would be without the herbs they traditionally include! Enriching the majority of our foods and beverages, herbs are another proof of how fully God provides for us—even in the small details of life!

Although their first use is in cooking, most culinary herbs do well in the medicinal realm too—making it hard to categorize some of them! As you will notice, there's a fine line between culinary and medicinal for several of the upcoming herbs. The good part is that nearly all culinary herbs are high in vitamins, minerals, and properties that promote overall health. So go ahead and make frequent use of your culinary herb collection. They aren't just tasty; they're a healthy addition to your favorite meal!

The following pages include brief profiles of fifteen enriching and delicious culinary herbs. If you aren't familiar with all of them, I encourage you to try those that are new to you. I think you'll enjoy the tasty experience!

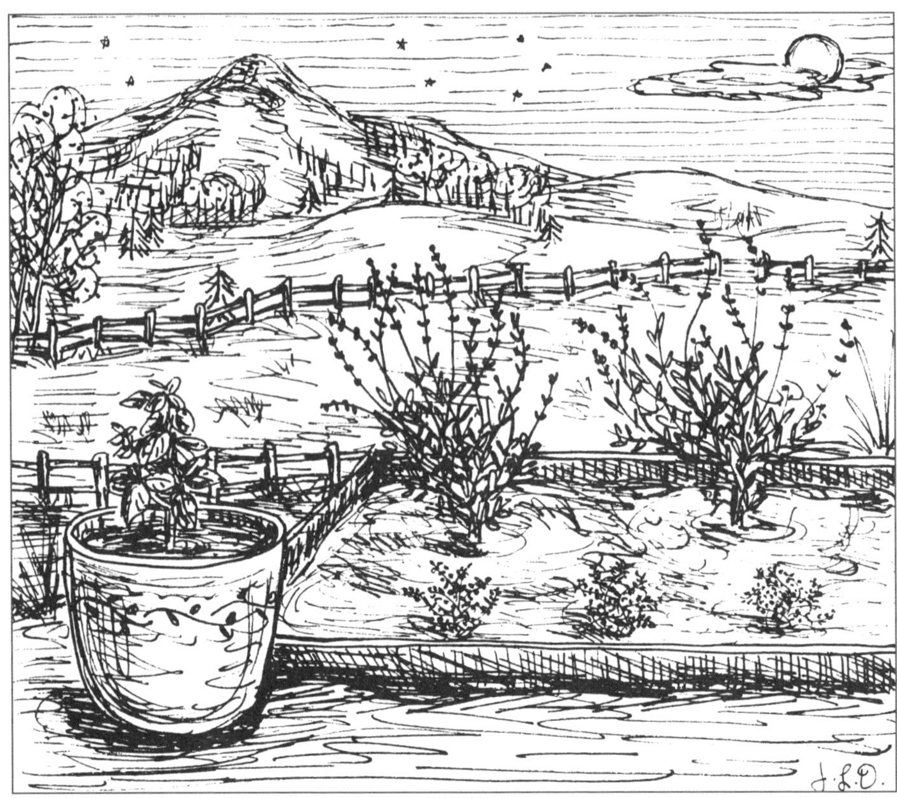

BASIL

Sweet basil, *Ocimum basilicum;* Bush basil, *O. basilicum* var. *minimum;* Lime basil, *O. basilicum* var. *americanum:* Labiatae family, annual.

It would seem to be simple to write about basil, one of the most-loved culinary herbs. However, it's harder than one might think! The many different varieties, each unique in its scent, flavor, growth habit, size, and shape, could fill an entire book devoted to basil alone. Since there are quite a few other herbs I'd like to showcase, I decided to narrow this one to three of my favorite varieties!

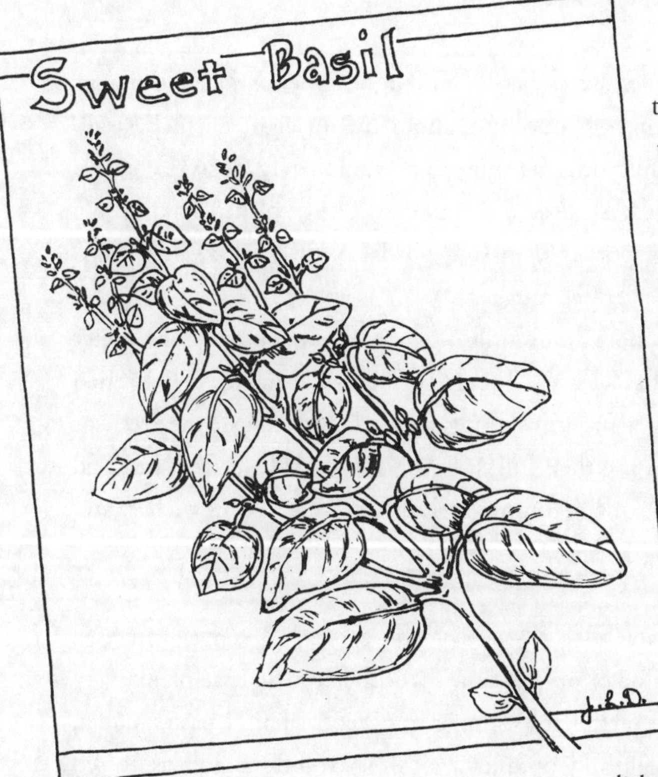

Sweet basil comes out at the top of the list, especially the "Sweet Genovese" strain. With broad, glossy, tender leaves that have a particularly pleasing taste, this variety is prized for its use in Greek and Italian dishes.

Blended with parsley, olive oil, garlic, Parmesan cheese, and pine nuts (or walnuts), the familiar pesto sauce is made. Sweet basil is also exceptional in nearly all tomato dishes, such as pizza sauce (along with oregano), tomato soup, and tomato-based stews. I like it dried and sprinkled liberally on garlic bread or over pasta, tossed fresh in leaf salads, and perking up egg or cheese dishes.

It is interesting to note that basil supports the digestive system, making it a welcome addition to the rich Greek and Italian dishes it complements so well. But don't limit sweet basil to these dishes—it goes well with many soups; in rice dishes; added to steamed carrots, cabbage, or spinach; baked with fish; and a number of other dishes. Try it sprinkled over slices of garden-fresh tomatoes and topped with a vinegar dressing. Yum!

Sweet basil grows about twenty inches high. It has broad, tender, wonderfully fragrant leaves and produces long spikes of white flowers that attract bees. A fragile herb that can't tolerate cold, I like to plant it with tomatoes in the greenhouse, or in a sunny spot on the deck. Harvest leaves above the second pair of leaves and pinch back flowers to promote a bushier plant.

Bush basil is hardier than sweet basil—and it bears a markedly different appearance! Shapely and compact (reaching about five to eighteen inches tall, depending on the type), many gardeners enjoy bush basil merely for its decorative appearance. Tiny scented leaves cover the rounded, bushy plant, making it a pretty sight when grown in pots, old mixing bowls, or, if it's a dwarf variety, chipped teapots and oversized coffee mugs.

Although sweet basil is most commonly used for pesto, some cooks prefer the unique flavor of bush basil leaves. The spicy, clove-like fragrance is carried over into the taste, making a mouthwatering pesto. Gently crush the fresh or dried leaves before use, releasing their fullest flavor. I like to blend fresh or dried leaves into cream cheese, making a yummy spread for crackers, sandwiches, and hamburgers.

Lime basil is somewhat rare, but seeds are available through Botanical Interests, Inc. (see page 223) This is one of our all-time favorite herbs that we plant every year. With appearance and growth habits similar to sweet basil, lime basil's tender, light green leaves have a delightfully unique flavor. It is exceptional in teas, tossed in salads, and so much more—including desserts like sorbet! Try it in pesto for a tastebud-tingling twist. And it is simply refreshing added to lemonade!

All three varieties grow easily from seed sown outdoors directly in warm soil. You can start seeds indoors six or eight weeks before the last spring frost, transferring to the garden when the soil is warm. But be very gentle, as the fragile little seedlings sometimes resent being transplanted. All prefer full sun and warm, well-drained, moist soil throughout the growing season. Frost and cold will quickly destroy these delicate plants, so be sure to protect them if a cold spell is expected.

All types of basil have medicinal value as well as culinary. Not only does basil (especially sweet basil) support the digestive system, it is also good for settling an upset stomach and relieving nausea. All varieties are bacteria- and fungus-fighting, and poultices of the fresh leaves can be helpful for treating acne, rashes, and even ringworm.

A handy way to preserve basil leaves is to lay them in a single layer on a baking sheet and place in the freezer. Once frozen, store in airtight containers in the freezer for several months. Other options are to prepare as pesto (omitting the cheese until thawed) and freeze. Olive oil takes on a murky appearance when frozen, but this doesn't affect the quality of the mixture. You may also chop the fresh leaves and blend them into softened butter; shape, place in freezer-safe containers, and freeze for several months.

The leaves dry quickly (and retain a good flavor!) if laid in a single layer on a screen and placed in a cool, dry, dark area for several days until crumbly. Store dry herbs in an airtight container.

Tips

Culinary and medicinal benefits aren't all this delicate herb is good for—it repels flies too, making an excellent potted herb for the deck or patio. Or why not scatter basil bouquets on your picnic table? Fresh or dried, flies avoid them!

In your garden or greenhouse, plant basil and marigolds among your tomatoes: they repel whiteflies and harmful soil nematodes, and help the tomatoes flourish. I do this and am pleased with the results!

BAY

"Noble laurel," "sweet bay" *(Laurus nobilis):* Lauraceae family, perennial. Zones 7–9.

What usually comes to mind when you think of herbs? For me, it's bushy little plants that fit easily into a small garden plot. With bay, such is not the case! A native to the Mediterranean (as are many herbs), this herb grows into a simply breathtaking 60-foot-tall evergreen tree in warm and mild climates. In cooler climates it reaches 25 feet, and in cold climates it makes a good potted tree if kept trimmed and moved into the greenhouse to overwinter.

Bay doesn't mind getting a trimming, so don't be afraid to use your pruning shears. In fact, bay trees are often used as ornamental shrubs and pruned into many shapes. When grown in containers, they must be kept well-trimmed to flourish. But if you've ever seen a full-sized tree, you might agree with me that bay is at its most beautiful with its gracefully branching natural shape!

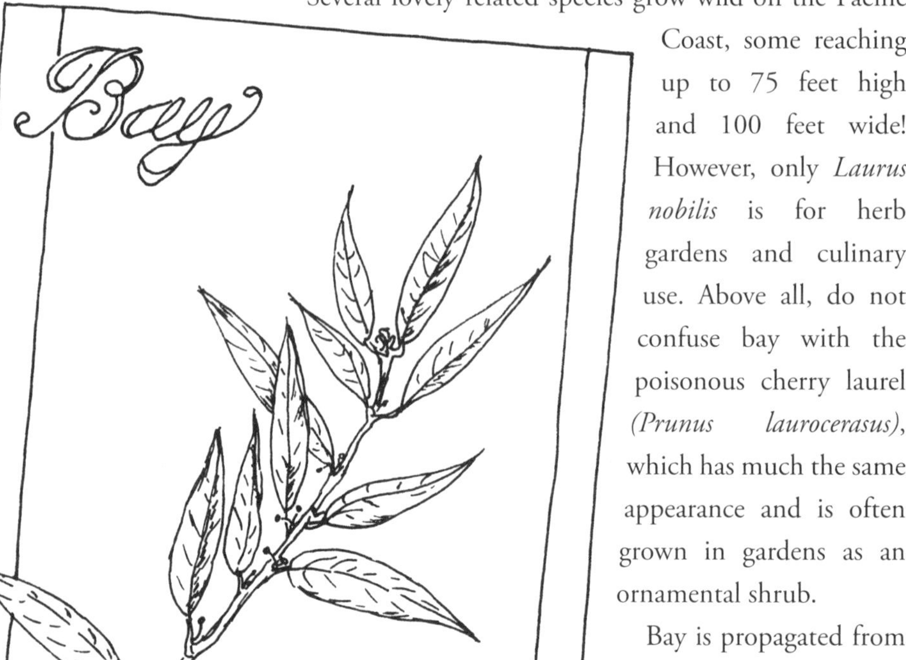

Several lovely related species grow wild on the Pacific Coast, some reaching up to 75 feet high and 100 feet wide! However, only *Laurus nobilis* is for herb gardens and culinary use. Above all, do not confuse bay with the poisonous cherry laurel *(Prunus laurocerasus)*, which has much the same appearance and is often grown in gardens as an ornamental shrub.

Bay is propagated from seed or rooted sucker cuttings. Both take months to become established, which (according to me!) makes purchasing a tree the best choice. Bay trees can stand brief temperatures as low as 30 degrees, but an extended freeze seals their fate: a slow but sure death. Plant in well-drained, sandy soil in a protected, partly sunny corner of your yard. Water regularly, misting the leaves occasionally. You may cut the trees into shrubs, cut the lower branches to make a topiary shape, or allow trees to grow into their natural form. Feed with a complete fertilizer each spring.

If your winters get consistently colder than 45 degrees, bay must be grown in a container and moved indoors when the cold season hits. Keep the tree trimmed and it will probably never grow larger than four feet tall. Use well-drained, sandy soil and be sure not to overwater or let it dry out completely. Mist the leaves frequently. In winter, place in a greenhouse or sunny window, keeping temperatures between 45 and 80 degrees. Keep soil barely moist. Feed in spring with a complete fertilizer and move outdoors as soon as the weather is favorable. Indoors, bay is an herb of choice for mealybugs, plus prone to scale. Wipe leaves with a cotton ball dipped in rubbing alcohol or horticultural oil. (Wash leaves before using!) In mild cases, you may try a mixture of dish soap, cooking oil, and warm water to kill the bugs. Add baking soda to the mixture for scale.

Harvest leaves at any time, using fresh or dried. To dry, lay on screens in a dark, dry, well-ventilated area. When dry, store whole leaves in an airtight container. Do not crush the leaves!

In late spring to midsummer, greenish white blossoms grace the bay tree. Bees love them! The flowers are followed by shiny purple-black berries that become hard when they dry. The deep green leaves are strong, leathery, and oblong, beautifully shiny on top, and pungently fragrant when bruised or torn. The leaves and berries both contain essential oil. Both oils are used for external medicinal purposes only, such as treating bruises, sprains, and sore, overused muscles; or diluted in water as a facial cleanser. Never take these oils internally! They contain dangerous narcotic properties.

Culinary use of bay leaves as seasoning, however, is safe—just don't eat the leaves! Fresh, their taste is stronger and just a little bitter. The dried leaves (which are sweeter in both flavor and aroma) are the traditional way to cook with bay. As mentioned, fresh or dried bay leaves are not to be ingested. Be sure to remove from dishes before serving!

If you have never used bay to season foods, start off with a very small amount—it is *strong!* Some describe the taste as "woodsy," some "spicy;" all agree that it is pungent. You may mellow the flavor by making a bouquet of fresh parsley stalks, thyme, marjoram, and one fresh bay leaf (one of the many variations of *bouquet garni*). Or add a few whole cloves along with bay leaf. On its own, you may tie half a leaf or more (fresh or dried) in cheesecloth and place in soups, stews, meat dishes, casseroles, fish, sea foods, pot roasts, and more while cooking, then remove leaves before serving. Bay imparts a unique and noticeable flavor that is said to enliven any meat dish. You might notice that the flavor goes especially well with lamb and fish, which are common dishes in the Mediterranean—not surprising, since that is home-sweet-home to bay trees!

Bay leaves may also be used to flavor marinades and tomato dishes, and are often found in pickling spice mixes.

Tip

Tuck a few dried bay leaves into bins of flour or grain, line your pantry shelves, and place in kitchen cupboards—the pungent aroma helps keep insects away!

> *Let us consider that we have a necessary dependence upon God for all the supports of this life. Our food comes all out of the earth, to remind us whence we ourselves were taken and whither we must return, and that therefore we must not think to live by bread alone, for that will feed the body only, but must look into the Word of God for the meat that endures to eternal life.*
>
> *–Matthew Henry on Psalm 104:14*

CARAWAY

(Carum carvi): Umbelliferae family, biennial. Zones 3–4.

Hmm, doesn't that lacy, delicate plant look a bit like dill or fennel? It certainly does! Meet a member of the Umbelliferae family. Like many families, Umbelliferaes usually resemble one another and share some of the same traits—but let me assure you that they are all *quite* uniquely individual!

Caraway likes a lot of sun, but otherwise it is one of the easiest herbs to grow. Freely reseeding if allowed to, this herb thrives in nearly any type of soil—even the worst! No wonder it can turn into a nuisance and is sometimes called a weed. But believe me, it's worth it to have a nice bed of caraway in your garden. The culinary and medicinal uses make it a favorite herb.

You may sow seed directly in the garden in the spring or fall. If planted in the fall, it will flower when summer comes. If planted in the spring, you may have to wait until the next year to see blossoms and harvest seeds. Add organic matter to your soil, rough up the surface, scatter seed, and pat down; in the spring keep moist—and wait. In about two weeks (once the soil is warm) little seedlings will pepper the ground.

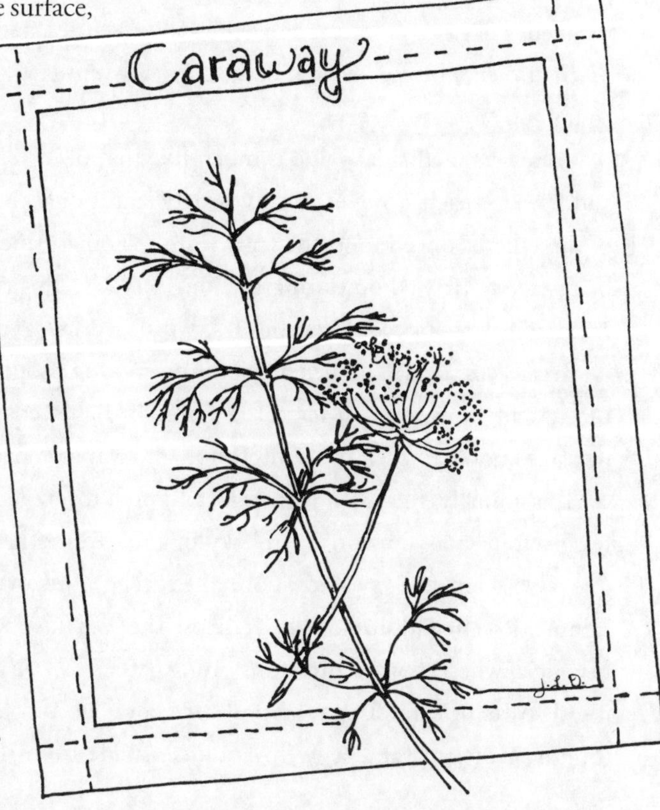

Caraway grows into two-foot-tall, slender (but sturdy) plants with long, divided, bright green feathery leaves that resemble carrot tops. In midsummer until sometime in September, attractive three- to four-inch umbels (flat-topped, rounded flower clusters) of tiny individual white or pink flowers (with an aroma resembling dill) make a lovely backdrop for shorter herbs. Caraway is typically a biennial, but, as mentioned previously, it will freely reseed and reappear in force early each spring. But don't let too many of the seeds fall! These are a valuable part of the plant.

The feathery young leaves may be harvested at any time during the growing season. They are used in soups and salads, or added to beets, spinach, or zucchini during the steaming process to impart a subtle, appetizing flavor. I like to incorporate the leaves into potato salads for a unique taste! The roots may be dug in late summer of the first year and cooked much like the vegetable they resemble—parsnips. You may want to sow a separate bed of caraway simply for the young, tender roots. The dried seeds, however, are what I consider the best part of caraway! Wait until the flowers are spent, then cut off the heads. Keep in single layers on paper-towel-lined baking sheets on your kitchen counter (preferably with a nice cross-breeze from open windows), and move to catch the sun. Once the seeds fall easily from the flowerheads (now dried and shriveled), let them dry on their own a bit longer in a dark, dry, well-ventilated area. Store in an airtight container.

Caraway's medicinal value is much like that of its family members anise, dill, and fennel—each being especially beneficial for digestive health. The seeds of all of these herbs once found their way into Colonial American meeting houses, to be discreetly chewed on during the long services. This calmed hunger pangs and eased embarrassing stomach noises. Try it! It works.

Because caraway is so beneficial for promoting proper digestion and cleansing the system, consuming a few of the protein-rich seeds daily (best taken with a meal) is known to clear the complexion and improve overall health.

Traditionally, the seeds were infused into a tea, cooled, then strained and the tea given in small portions to colicky infants. To soothe an upset stomach, crush one tablespoon caraway seeds, pour one cup hot milk over them, and steep for ten minutes. Strain and sip slowly—it helps! The seeds also sweeten the breath and are beneficial when chewed after consuming garlic.

All parts of caraway are helpful for glandular and kidney health. It also has topical medicinal value as well. Poultices made from the seeds are excellent for treating bruises, while infusions added to complexion soaps or used as a rinse are both cleansing and soothing.

With amazing medicinal value, caraway is a good choice for your medicinal herb garden. But wait until you hear about its culinary uses! Healthful enough to be considered "medicinal food," it is also a most delicious wonder—from head to foot! That is why I eagerly put caraway in the culinary section.

Caraway seeds are mouthwateringly aromatic and have a spicy, lingering warm taste that is just a little like lemon peel. Remember how I mentioned that they are a valuable part of the plant? Considering their many uses, I know you'll agree!

Whenever I taste or smell caraway seeds, I automatically think of rye bread or those delicious crackers seasoned with caraway seed and so perfect for topping with sharp cheddar cheese. Try sprinkling a few seeds in your next grilled cheese sandwich before grilling—you'll thank me for the yummy suggestion! And the seeds are wonderful in just about any baked goods. Who can resist caraway crackers, biscuits, bread, or delightful caraway biscotti alongside a cup of hot tea? I like to add a sprinkle of seeds to the batter of cakes and scones, spreading the just-out-of-the-oven treats with strawberry jam. When baking apples or pears, follow your favorite recipe and sprinkle with a few caraway seeds before baking. They can also be added to applesauce recipes for a delicious (and healthful!) difference.

Caraway seeds are a part of many sauerkraut recipes and also many delicious cheese recipes. To quickly try their flavor in cheese, add to cream cheese (refrigerate for at least 24 hours so the flavors will blend) for a tasty spread! Or make traditional Scottish "crowdie," a dish using curds and caraway—basically cottage cheese with caraway seeds and ground black pepper mixed in (left in the refrigerator for a day or two to blend flavors) and served sprinkled with salt. This makes a great lunch teamed up with whole wheat crackers, a tossed salad, and a glass of salted tomato juice!

The fresh leaves add a tang to salads (remember, try them in potato salad!) and soups, while the roots are rather sweet and a bit earthy in flavor, perfect served with butter or gravy.

Caraway seeds and leaves go well with onion and potato dishes too. Combine and boil until tender, then serve with butter. You can add a few caraway roots if you'd like. Luscious! The seeds and fresh leaves are also excellent when added during the steaming process of beets, carrots, cabbage, or cauliflower.

Considering its varied uses in the kitchen, why not add this wonderful, low-maintenance herb to your garden?

Tips

Caraway may resemble its Umbelliferae family members, but none of them prefer to live near one another. In fact, if planted nearby, they will hinder each other's growth!

Plant caraway in that poor-soil section of your yard—the roots loosen heavy soil and help improve the overall condition.

CHIVES

(Allium schoenoprasum): Lilaceae family, perennial. Zones 3–10.

What do you usually look for as being the "first herald of spring"? Some might say apple blossoms or daffodils, but for me it's—chives! When the first drying winds come to lick up the snow here in the Rockies, I step outside and check on my snowcapped barrels of chives. I already know what to expect: small, bright green needles of brave, cold-hardy leaves pricking through the snow! What a thrill for the gardener, getting them itching to work in the warm, fragrant earth again and enjoy the unbeatable quality of fresh herbs and vegetables! But of course, for me the sight of chives is just a hint of what is to come…*later.* With our frost-free period only about 82 days, I know I can't expect to work the soil until early June. So I smile a welcome to the chives and hurry back indoors to get out of the cold!

Chives are perhaps the least troublesome herb to grow. Most pests (insects, rodents, and deer) are usually repelled by them, allowing them to grow in peace. Interplanting among vegetables and other herbs often keeps pests away from those plants as well! And chives aren't invasive, so you don't have to worry about them taking over where they don't belong.

In cold locations, a good trimming in the fall makes their dormant winter sleep more profitable, and they wake up bright, early, and vigorous in the spring. Don't discard the fall trimmings, though! Preserve them for winter use.

Although chives prefer cool temperatures (below 75 degrees), they are very accommodating to location and act as evergreens in the South. Creation can illustrate many lessons for us, and I always think of chives as a good example of showing contentment in whatever state we are in! Sun or partial shade, damp or dry soil that's either rich or poor, containers, borders, or beds—chives usually flourish contentedly. However, they won't resent slightly acid, moderately rich soil, several applications of all-purpose fertilizer, and consistent watering!

Chives are a clump-forming herb in the onion family. At a glance, they may appear to be a humble clump of grass. Take a closer look! The hollow, sturdy leaves grow to be about ten inches tall and form small bulbs (similar to scallions) just under the ground. Pinch off a leaf and breathe deeply. The onion-like scent is deliciously appetizing, and if you chew on a piece you'll notice the mild, fresh flavor permeating your mouth. (You may want to pluck a sprig of parsley to chew on after that—it will sweeten your breath!) Pinkish-lavender globe-shaped flowerheads make a pretty sight when allowed to bloom.

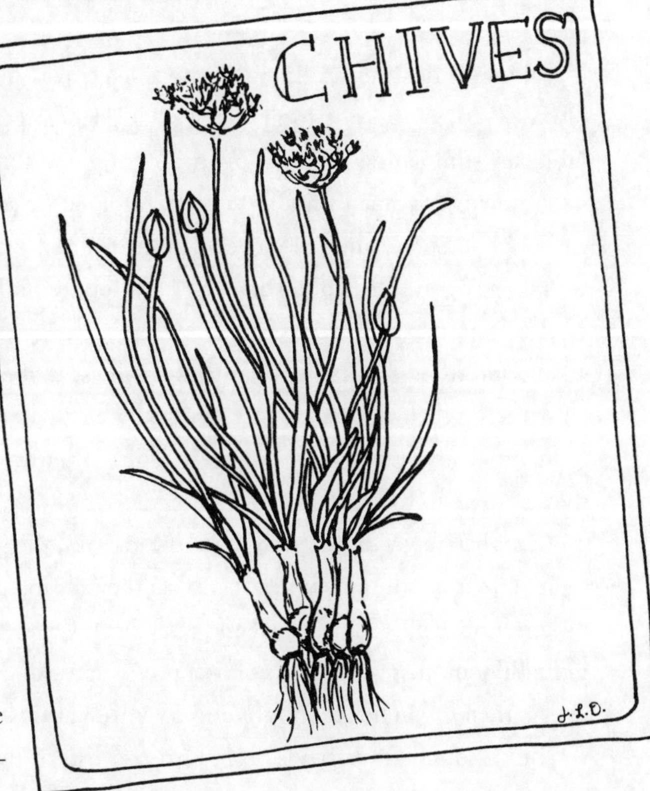

Every part is edible, but the hollow leaves are especially tasty. Chives—

like grass—are kept healthy by regular trimming. We don't consider that a problem, since we use large quantities of fresh-snipped chives throughout the growing season! This promotes new growth—above ground where new leaves come, and below ground where new bulbs form. Since chives grow in clumps, they may be separated in the spring or fall every three or four years. It takes about six clumps of chives to keep a family of six happy.

To preserve chives for winter use, chop fresh chives finely and mix with a very little bit of water. Spoon into ice cube trays reserved for this purpose (they'll taste like chives ever-afterwards!) and freeze. Remove from trays to freezer containers. This method best preserves the flavor. When needed, simply thaw an ice cube in a shallow bowl, strain, and then gently squeeze chives dry in a paper towel.

For drying chives, I suggest snipping the fresh chives finely and spreading them in a single layer on a paper-towel-lined baking sheet. Drape a piece of cheesecloth over the baking sheet and put in a cool, dry, dark place for about a week (stirring twice a day) or until thoroughly dry. Store in an airtight container in a dark, cool place.

Falling under the "culinary herb" title, chives have limited medicinal use. However, they are nutritious as well as delicious, containing vitamins and minerals, stimulating healthy appetite, acting as a tonic on the kidneys, and are said to help (in a small way) to lower high blood pressure.

In the kitchen, snipped chives—fresh or dried—are delicious anywhere you would use onions. The bulbs may be used too, reminiscent of green onions. Top a baked potato, stir into rice, scramble up with eggs, sprinkle over tacos, toss in salads, add to dips and cheese spreads—the list is almost limitless! Be aware that chives are at their ultimate best fresh, and are still good dried, but they lose most of their flavor when cooked. I suggest adding after the cooking process, or during the last three to five minutes of cooking.

But what about those lovely flowerheads? Yes, they are more than just a pretty sight! Pinch off the flowerheads just as they are blooming and sauté lightly in butter or olive oil—an unusual and tasty treat! Or use the edible lavender flowers in full bloom, tossed in salads or as a pretty garnish. Some like to dip the flowers in egg, then roll in bread crumbs and fry until lightly browned. I haven't tried that yet, but it sounds so tasty it's on my "to-try" list for this summer!

Chives make a hassle-free addition to any herb garden and add a perky flavor to most foods. If your garden doesn't include them yet, maybe that should be on *your* "to-try" list come spring!

Tips

In the garden, chives seem to have a beneficial effect on carrots when grown alongside them. They also make a pest-deterring border around your herb and vegetable gardens!

Note: Garlic chives, or "Chinese chives" *(Allium tuberosum),* have a distinct garlic/chive flavor that is characteristic of Oriental dishes. These chives have flat leaves and are strongly reminiscent of garlic in taste and smell. They are a nice variation to common chives, both in the garden and in the kitchen!

CORIANDER/CILANTRO

"Chinese Parsley" *(Coriandrum sativum):* Umbelliferae family, annual.

Welcome to another member of the Umbelliferae family, coriander/cilantro. No, that's not a typo! This one plant combines two wonderful taste adventures, making up my all-time favorite culinary herb(s)! And on a warm summer day, no matter where I'm at in the yard, I can tell if someone has brushed against the delicate leaves or plucked and chewed on a seed (technically fruit) in the herb garden. The unique, powerful scent of both the leaves and fruit is wafted deliciously on the breeze!

Despite its culinary wonder, the plant itself isn't exactly impressive. It's spindly (reaching about 2½ feet on a few branched stems) and might need staking to keep it from sprawling over in a tangled heap. The lower leaves, divided into broad segments, and the delicate, feathery upper leaves of the plant are both known as cilantro (sometimes called Chinese parsley). Their pungent, fresh lemony scent and flavor is wonderful once you get used to it! When allowed to flower, cilantro has small, light pink umbels that add delicate charm to the tall, feathery plant—and strongly attract honeybees! When the large seeds (technically fruits) form, they are known as coriander—and are a whole different story from cilantro! Their aroma and flavor is exceedingly strong when green, but becomes spicy-sweet as they ripen and dry. Let them mature to a golden brown, then gently rub from the stems. You will find yourself breathing deeply of the warm, spicy scent that is reminiscent of citrus and sage, mixed with a hint of anise. I like to eat the mature seeds whole, right off the plant.

This exceptional annual is easy to grow. I suggest having one patch devoted to the leaves and one to the fruit. Direct-seed in mid-spring after the last frost, or scatter seed in the fall. Average, well-drained soil is good, and be sure to water consistently.

For your cilantro patch, make sure there's partial shade (to help prevent bolting) and keep the soil moist (but not wet). Pinch out flower stalks as they form. It's helpful to use an all-purpose, water-soluble fertilizer at least twice a month to promote lush foliage. Miracle-Gro™ works well for me.

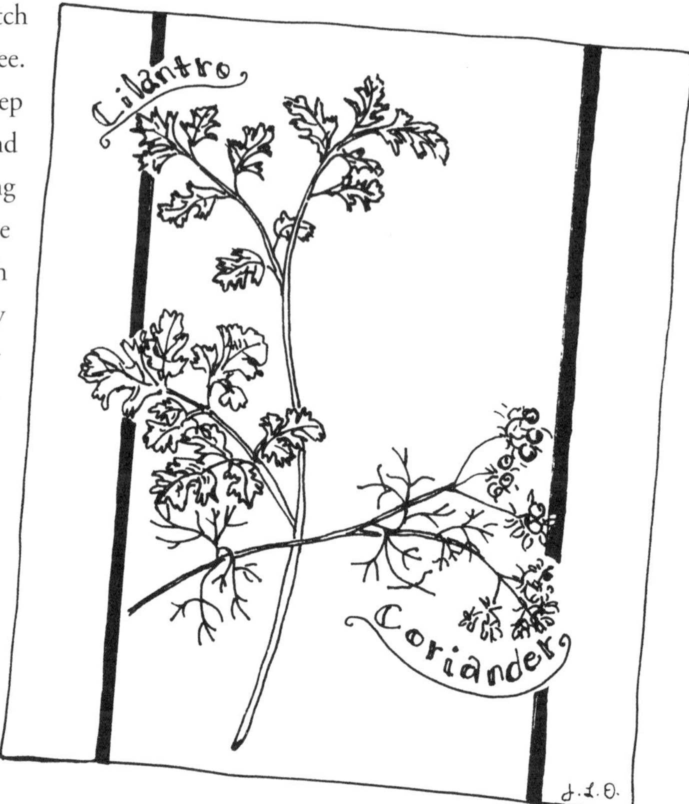

Your coriander patch is a bit more carefree. Plant in full sun, keep the soil rather dry, and soon you'll be harvesting seeds! Oh, and be sure to set aside enough seeds to replant every two weeks for a steady supply of greenery over in your cilantro patch!

Although viewed as a culinary herb, both cilantro and coriander (but especially coriander!) contain medicinal value too. Cilantro contains vitamins A and C and important minerals (calcium, phosphorus, potassium, and iron). Coriander is excellent for promoting digestive health. Eating a few seeds after a meal is beneficial, or including them *in* parts of the meal is even better! The seeds used to be prescribed for kidney stones and urinary troubles. One caution: don't overdo it! Excessively high amounts of the seeds can be narcotic, and an overdose of the juice of fresh cilantro is dangerous.

Cilantro does not dry well, so it's best used fresh-picked. Go ahead and dry some, though, if you prefer a more mild flavor! You may also freeze finely chopped cilantro in a bit of water in ice cube trays; but it, too, loses some of that powerful punch. Coriander seeds (or fruits) should be harvested when they are a golden brown. After harvesting, allow them to dry thoroughly in a cool, dry, dark place, then store in an airtight container.

Now let's step into the kitchen! Cilantro's pungent flavor is unbeatable in salsa, cream cheese spreads, green salads, rice dishes, and many ethnic cuisines, especially Chinese and Mexican cooking. Cilantro was an integrated part of growing up in southern California, where the herb is prevalent in local cooking. Even here in southwest Colorado, it is commonly used. But be warned! If you have never cooked with cilantro, its strong aroma and unique taste may take some getting used to. Start out using small amounts in tomato- or avocado-based dishes, since its flavor is at its exceptional best with these. Cilantro is also tasty added to sauces, or (sparingly) steeped along with green tea. The frost-work of greenery makes a lovely garnish too!

From sweet breads to savory stews, coriander is quite versatile! And remember, the flavor is comparable to what manna tasted like! (Exodus 16:31.) A pinch of the finely ground seed is tasty in fish, poultry, and meat dishes. Coriander is also a part of traditional curry, lending its warmly sweet flavor. Or how about adding a bit to a shaker of ground black pepper and sprinkling over pork roasts or other meat dishes for a gentle, pleasant, spicy-sweet taste? Combine a few whole dried seeds with your bread and butter pickling blend—delicious! My favorite use of coriander, however, is adding the finely ground seeds to spice cakes, corn breads, yeast breads, pastries, and apple or peach desserts. Try it! The yummy result is hard to beat. And it's a healthy addition too!

Does your herb garden include this exceptional two-in-one herb? If not, I highly recommend incorporating it in your next planting!

Tips

Coriander/cilantro doesn't seem to mind being crowded together. In fact, I suggest planting a bed of this herb with each plant only about eight or nine inches apart. Then they can help hold each other up!

Incorporate anise into your coriander/cilantro bed, or plant beds of each side-by-side. They seem to encourage healthy growth in one another. However, other Umbelliferae members seem to do the opposite, so keep them far away!

DILL

(Anethum graveolens): Umbelliferae family, annual.

Are you new at herb gardening and looking for a good plant to start with? Try dill! It was one of the first herbs I planted in my first herb garden, endearing itself to me by growing beautifully and being diversely useful! If you're a tried-and-true herb gardener, you are probably already familiar with this easy-to-grow, easy-to-harvest, and easy-to-preserve herb. It's also a pretty sight, plus it offers a few medicinal and many culinary uses—what could be better! Oh yes, and dill is yet another member of that large and wonderful Umbelliferae family.

Dill likes moderately rich, well-drained soil and full sun. After sowing the seeds, keep moist until they germinate in about ten to twenty days, then water moderately. In warmer climates, direct-sow as soon as the ground can be worked in the spring. Since dill needs a soil temperature of about 60 degrees to germinate, you will have to start sometime in late May or early June if your climate is cold. Dill takes about two months after germination to go through its growing cycle and produce seeds. But in warm climates don't harvest some of the flowerheads—they'll self-sow and give you a constant summer supply of fresh dill in the garden!

When dill comes into flower, it is a lovely sight—a burst of pale yellowish-green flowers cover the umbels that top the tall stalks. I suggest planting a patch of dill rather close together (about eight inches apart), so that the spindly plants will help hold each other up. They grow to about three feet tall, so don't place them where they will shade other sun-loving plants. You may plant them in deep containers with good drainage holes too, making a nice potted herb for your patio. Contrary to typical growing suggestions, I like to group dill, chives, and sweet basil in one large container, and it works beautifully too!

To harvest dillweed (the young, feathery foliage), do so sparingly from each plant so as not to destroy them. These are best used fresh and keep for about three or four days in the refrigerator, or about two months frozen (with a sprinkle of water added) in sealed containers. You may also dry dillweed, which is best done by laying whole sprigs of leaves on screens, then brushing off the dried leaves into airtight containers and discarding the stalks.

For pickling uses, snip off the whole flowerhead while still partially blooming and containing green seeds. This can go directly into your pickle jars. Dill seeds are gathered by harvesting the flowerheads just as the flowers are spent. Lay in single layers on paper-towel-lined baking sheets on your kitchen counter, preferably with a cross-breeze and lots of sun. When the flowerheads are dry and shriveled, gently shake out the dry seeds. Once thoroughly dry, store in an airtight container.

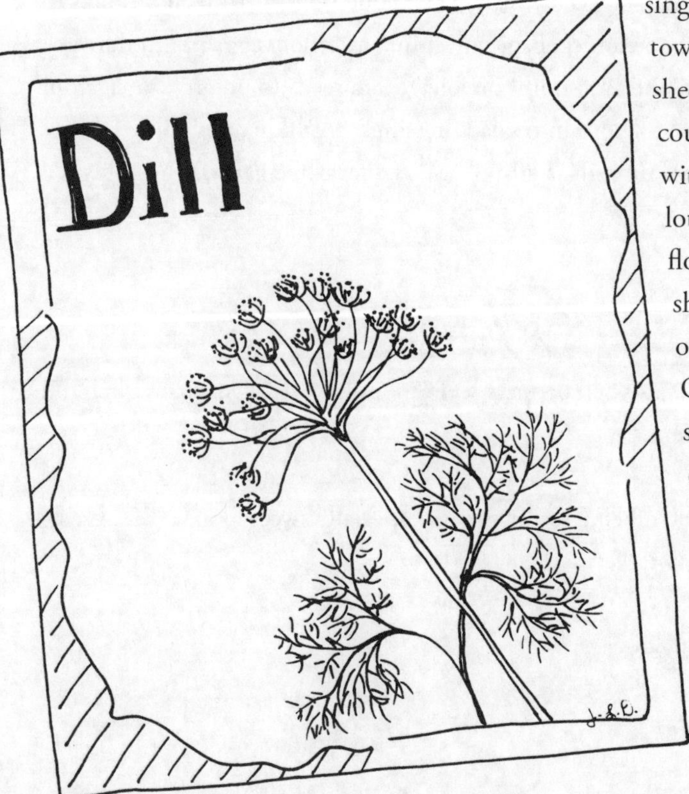

In the medicinal field, dill (especially the seed) has properties much like its Umbelliferae cousins anise, sweet fennel, and caraway. All are especially useful for treating digestive disorders and maintaining a healthy digestive tract. Dillweed and seeds are also good for relieving stomach flu symptoms, or used as a quick rescue from a bad case of hiccups! Chew a few dill leaves or seeds (the leaves have a milder, slightly anise taste, but don't contain as much of the beneficial oils as the seeds) after a meal to help food assimilation and to promote digestion.

In the culinary field, dill is considered a "medicinal food," promoting overall health by keeping the digestive tract in good shape. I personally think that dill pickles are the best and most delicious use for dill, making a tasty snack no matter what—and adding wonderfully to sandwiches and burgers. But dill (whether seed or weed) complements many dishes, such as soups, borscht, egg dishes, baked goods, and more! As mentioned previously, it's great in pickling spices, but also excellent added to vinegar, marinades, sauerkraut, sour cream-based dips, etc. Mix some dillweed in your egg salad for flavorful sandwiches! Sprinkle liberally over fried eggs and potatoes. Top tomato soup, stir into sauces for seafoods, and boil with potatoes. Dillweed is especially tasty when added the last fifteen minutes to baking or steaming fish. Steam cabbage, zucchini, and root veggies with dillweed too—the flavor is excellent. Add both the foliage and seeds to potato or macaroni salads for a perky flair. Mix both into salad dressings. Sprinkle dried dillweed over buttered vegetables, toss fresh in salads, or use as a fern-like garnish. Yes, this is a versatile herb!

Tips

Strawberries, tomatoes, and bell peppers seem to grow more vigorously when dill is interplanted with them.

Don't plant near other Umbelliferae members, especially sweet fennel. They cross-fertilize and hinder growth.

Dill flowers attract honeybees.

FENNEL

(Foeniculum vulgare): Umbelliferae family, biennial. Zones 6–9.

"What is that tall, feathery plant with big umbels of yellow flowers? It looks like a larger version of dill."

Yes, fennel does appear that way—but don't be fooled! Although they are in the same family (those Umbelliferaes again!), each is quite unique. After you taste and smell fennel, you'll think twice before substituting this powerful herb in your dill pickle recipe!

In temperate climates, fennel is a perennial and can reach the stunning height of seven feet. In cooler areas, it acts as a biennial and is a bit smaller in stature, not reaching its full potential until the second year. It has large, succulent, hollow stalks, feathery foliage that makes a pretty border (like a cloud of frothy green), and umbels of flowerheads that look much like dill when it flowers. Fennel boasts a myriad of uses— both culinary and medicinal. That's why it made my "Top Fifteen Favorite Herbs" list!

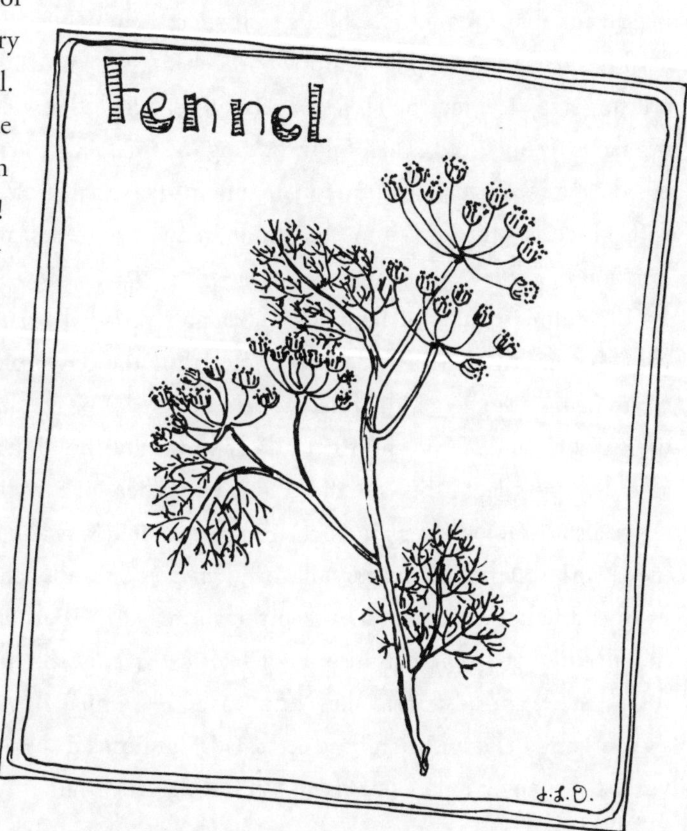

Fennel is easy to grow and does well from seed. Sow directly in rich garden soil in the fall or spring. Since fennel is a perennial in temperate climates and a biennial in cooler areas, you can divide the clump-forming plants in the spring. Fennel self-seeds freely, saving the trouble of sowing in the fall for next summer's garden! There is one drawback to the abundance of self-seeding, though—you will have to thin your fennel patch regularly to keep it from becoming weedy during the summer.

This herb grows nicely when placed against a fence or divider in your herb garden and given plenty of space. It prefers rich, warm soil, full sun, and moderate amounts of water. Harvest the feathery leaves as soon as they are big enough. Collect and dry seeds as you would dill seeds (see dill section). The stalks should be harvested while young and tender. To preserve, thoroughly dry all parts of fennel and store separately (seeds, stalks, and leaves) in airtight containers.

As with most chiefly culinary herbs, medicinal value is present and shouldn't be ignored. One of the most well-known medicinal uses of fennel leaves is for tired or inflamed eyes. Boil leaves in water for fifteen minutes, dip a soft cloth in the infused water, wring out excess water, and drape warm cloth over eyes. Repeat for about ten minutes. This really does help! Chewing a few seeds after a meal freshens the breath and improves digestion. Or make an after-dinner tea by bruising and steeping the leaves or seeds to enhance digestion and soothe upset stomachs. Fennel seed is helpful in ridding the intestinal tract of mucus and may be added to your daily routine to maintain intestinal health. Many attest that fennel increases the flow of mother's milk, reduces wrinkles, and promotes proper function of kidneys, liver, and spleen.

The culinary value of fennel is unbeatable. Loaded with nutrients, cooking with this healthful herb is a good choice! But the flavor alone would make it worth using. I suggest adding the seeds to rye breads or whole wheat dinner rolls, meat dishes, and stews, and the feathery leaves and hollow stalks to fish, cheese spreads, and salads—but go ahead and try either in any dish mentioned! The leaves also complement plain yogurt, making a delicious and nutritious snack, or blend with softened butter for a flavorful cracker or sandwich spread.

The dried seeds of fennel are my favorite part. They have a warm, sharp, mouthwatering flavor reminiscent of licorice or aniseed, complementing meat dishes, stews, breads, and cakes. The leaves are similar in taste (only just a bit sweeter) and delicious fresh in tossed salads, hummus dishes, and (as mentioned) yogurt. When the flat umbels of yellow flowers begin to bloom, snip some flowerheads off and add to leaf or fruit salads for a pretty (and tasty!) variation. The young peeled stalks are also flavorful and used in marinated salads, or dried and added to the roasting pan to gently season pork, fish, or chicken. In fact, this cooking procedure is said to help eliminate the oiliness of fish. The young, bright green stalks make a nice drinking straw, and are a good inducement to get children to drink cold vegetable smoothies. You might even want to try it yourself!

Caution: If you enjoy gathering wild herbs, don't try for fennel! In the wild it closely resembles poison hemlock, a deadly poisonous plant. If you want fennel, it's best to harvest only from plants that are ***absolutely known*** to be fennel!

Tips

Do not plant fennel near dill, cilantro, tomatoes, or beans—they aren't on friendly terms!

Fennel repels fleas.

Note: Many folks accidentally confuse fennel with its cousin Florence fennel (also called finocchio, *Foeniculum vulgare* var. *dulce).* Florence fennel acts more like a vegetable than an herb (although the leaves and seeds can be substituted for fennel, having similar medicinal and culinary value). It is mainly grown for its broad, tender leaf stalks and the large, crisp bulb that forms at the base of the plant. The flavor is delicate, sweet, and slightly anise—delicious cooked or raw. Why not sow a row in your garden?

FRENCH TARRAGON

(Artemisia dracunculus var. *sativa):* Compositae family, perennial. Zones 4–5.

With few medicinal properties, and yet so many taste-tingling uses in the kitchen, French tarragon comfortably settled into the culinary section!

French tarragon is sometimes confused with its near relation, Russian tarragon (simply *A. dracunculus*), but the two plants—though very similar in appearance—have at least two major differences: Russian tarragon is far inferior to French in flavor (you must use at least twice as much to get similar results); and French tarragon never produces seed, while Russian is easily propagated by seed.

The similarities of these two plants can cause a bit of confusion when looking to purchase true French tarragon, the cook's choice for ultimate tarragon flavor. Look closely for the botanical name, which will be *Artemisia dracunculus* var. *sativa*. Even then, be sure to ask permission to take a leaf, crush it to check the scent (which should be strongly licorice), and then chew on it. If it's true French tarragon, you'll get a burst of sharp licorice/mint flavor that lingers warmly in your mouth. When you come across seed packets simply marked "Tarragon," know, of course, that those are Russian tarragon seeds—certainly not French! Another good solution for securing a true plant for your garden is to check with friends and neighbors. Since French tarragon is propagated by

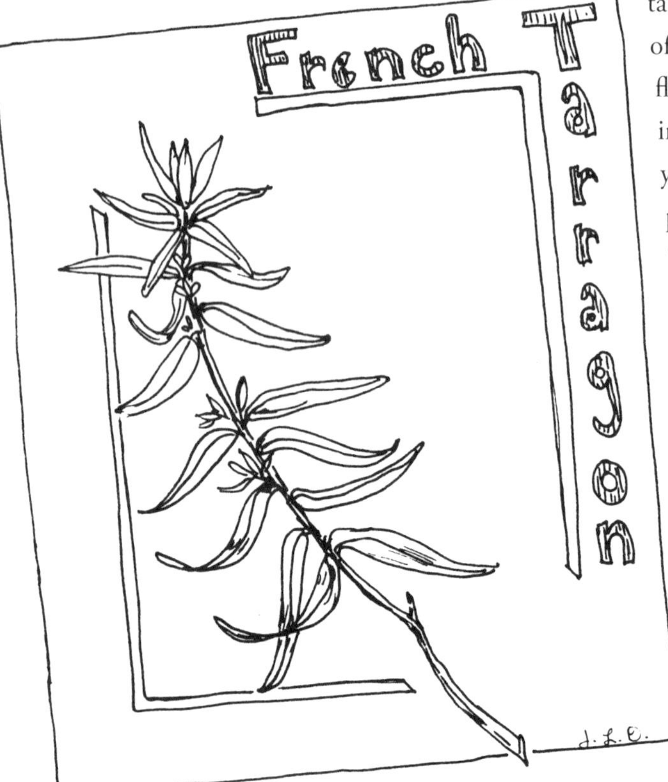

layering, tip cuttings, or simply root division, if someone has a tried-and-true plant, ask if you may take from that.

Once you have a real French tarragon plant established in your garden, take heart! True, it's only at its best for three or four years, but don't worry. The hardy perennial will grow into a sprawling bush that needs to be divided every two years, keeping you with a fresh supply of new plants. If you keep propagating when needed, your first plant will (through its successors) provide you with years and years of delicious French tarragon.

For a healthy plant, the soil needs to be well-drained (it's highly susceptible to root rot) and moderately rich. Add some sand and/or perlite for proper drainage. Make sure your planting site has the benefit of full sun, but is protected from wind. Keep in mind, too, that tarragon is drought-tolerant and doesn't require lots of water. If grown in a container, allow the soil to dry between watering. French tarragon likes cool, dry weather—it will quickly shrivel in hot, humid climates.

Space plants about a foot apart when planting, and a nice trimming in the summer (just as the small green flowers form) will encourage lush growth. In the fall, cut back nearly to the ground and, after the first hard frost, mulch heavily to encourage the needed dormant season and protect from harsh weather. In the spring, wait until you see little shoots of new growth and then rake away the mulch.

French tarragon also makes a nice container herb, being especially lovely (and convenient!) planted in a large barrel with thyme and savory. Some suggest overwintering tarragon in the house or greenhouse, but to do so risks the quality of the plant's strength and flavor. Going through a dormant season is important for keeping this herb vigorous.

The narrow, pointed dark green leaves are shiny and smooth. These are what you want for culinary use, and they're best picked in the morning and used fresh. However, if you like a milder tarragon flavor you may hang bunches (or lay in a single layer on a screen) in a cool, dry, dark, well-ventilated area and dry until crumbly. Store in an airtight container. To keep the bold flavor intact, you may also preserve tarragon in vinegar or infused oil. Then simply strain out a few leaves when you need them, and use as you would fresh tarragon (the vinegar and oil may be used in cooking too). Freezing in a bit of water in ice cube trays, then placing in airtight containers in the freezer also maintains much of the fresh flavor. Or if you like, you may blend with butter (a delicious combination, by the way!), shape, and freeze in sealed containers.

In the kitchen, it's easy to find many dishes to incorporate this sharp, tasty herb into. I find the flavor especially good with seafood when added to the dish itself, and/or served in tartar sauce alongside. And it complements other herbs too, such as garlic, parsley, and chives—which make a delightful mix sprinkled (fresh and finely minced) over baked potatoes, or (fresh or dried) for topping garlic bread! French tarragon delicately flavors meat and poultry, makes chicken or turkey soup a special treat, and lends flair to salads, pickles, and mustard. Try sautéing some tarragon in butter or olive oil, and then baste meat or poultry with it—the result is delicious. Steam some with sliced beets and cover with melted butter, making a wonderful flavor combination. Tarragon is also appetizing with egg and/or cheese dishes, such as quiches. Or blend into sour cream or mayonnaise. Tarragon complements dressings and white sauces too.

Are you hungry now, after reading all of that? I hope it encourages you to search out a true French tarragon plant for your garden—or, if you already have one, to make more use of it!

Tip

French tarragon is delightfully aromatic, and is a welcome neighbor to most other plants.

Note: Mexican tarragon *(Tagetes lucida),* also called winter tarragon, is actually a perennial marigold that thrives in hot climates. The leaves taste markedly like French tarragon, and yes, they can be used as a substitute! The bright yellow flowers of Mexican tarragon set seed, so it's a worthwhile addition to your garden—especially if you live where it is too hot for French tarragon to thrive.

GARLIC

(Allium sativum): Liliaceae family, perennial. Zones 2–10.

I blush to admit that for many years I never thought of garlic as an herb. It was just another plant in the vegetable garden, kind of like a root veggie, right? Wrong! Since it's in the genus *Allium,* along with chives, you might chuckle at my ignorance. In fact, many species of the genus *Allium* (onions, shallots, etc.) are considered both culinary and medicinal herbs. But I never stopped to think of it!

Garlic is featured in many herb books as one of the most beneficial of all medicinal herbs. At the same time, it holds a staggering degree of popularity in every nation's cuisine, complementing nearly any dish you can imagine. And the flavor—unique, pungent, appetizing—is exceptional, so even if you prefer only a touch of garlic at first, it will probably grow on you and you'll find yourself increasing the amount. Go ahead! Even when it is cooked, garlic retains its medicinal value, making it healthful as well as delicious! That's why I chose to put this versatile herb in the culinary category.

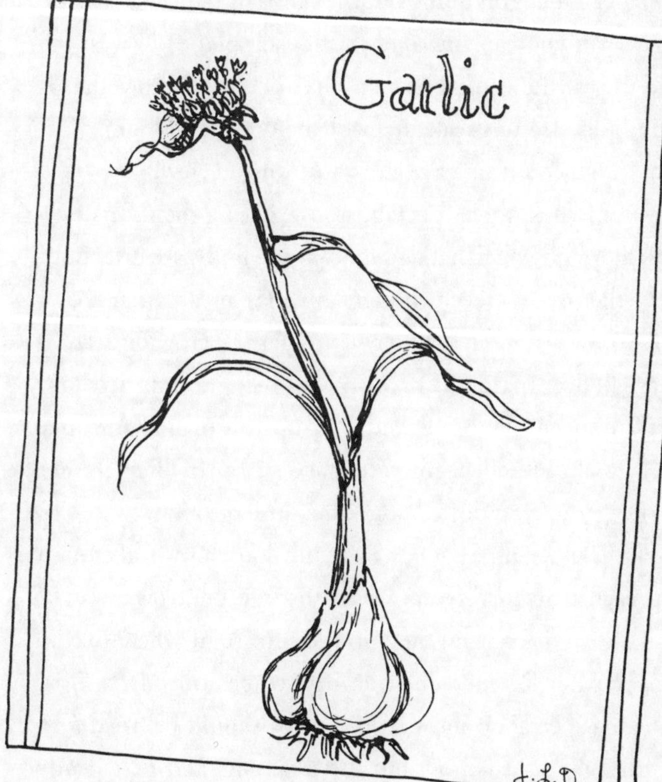

Garlic is easy and fun to grow. But be aware that it takes at least six months to mature. The bulb is divided into eight to twenty segmented cloves, covered with translucent papery white or pinkish skin. Separate these cloves, which are considered the "seed" for growing garlic. Plant the largest cloves for satisfactory results. Garlic requires full sun and ample water to thrive. In deeply dug, rich, well-drained soil, plant individual cloves about two inches deep (with the pointed end up!) and five inches apart. It may help to have the points just barely peeking out of the ground, or only lightly covered if you plant in the spring. Planting cloves in the fall seems to be the best choice, though, since garlic takes a *long* time to mature. If put into the ground about five or six weeks before the soil freezes in the fall, you can expect far better results when it comes time to harvest the bulbs in the upcoming late July or early August. Be sure to mulch well as soon as the ground freezes, and then in early spring rake back the mulch and begin a steady watering schedule. In late spring it's beneficial to treat with liquid seaweed extract to encourage growth.

Garlic likes cool weather to get established, which is another reason why planting in the fall is a good idea. It gives the cloves a chance to get comfortable in their new home throughout the cold winter and cool spring. Then during the heat of the upcoming summer, it can focus on filling out the bulbs into nice, fat cloves. All through the growing season you can (*sparingly* from each plant!) harvest the flavorful green shoots and use as you would green onions or chives. If flowerheads form, it may increase the bulb size to break them off before they bloom. (But they're quite pretty, so you might want to leave a few just for the view!)

Once the plants are about two to three feet tall, stop watering them. In a few days the leaves will turn yellow and wilt. That's a sign that the bulbs are just about ready to harvest! To hurry the process (even though this may mean a harvest of smaller bulbs), knock the tops over about 100 days into garlic's growing season. A few days after the leaves fall over (naturally or with your help) and turn yellow, you may loosen the dirt around a few bulbs and pull up the plants. Are they segmented and fat? If so, go ahead and begin your harvest! But if they are not segmented, be patient. Your garlic crop needs more time underground.

When garlic bulbs are sufficiently large enough, carefully loosen the soil around them and gently pull up each plant. Everyone seems to have their own way of drying garlic! Some simply leave them lying there in the sun, right where they've pulled them up. Others say wash first and then let dry, while still others insist that this shortens storage life expectancy and that the bulbs should be dried *first,* and *then* the excess dirt carefully brushed off and the dry roots and tops gently removed. Some simply braid the tops of freshly dug garlic, and hang the bulbs to dry in a warm, dry, breezy area. Whatever your method of choice, it takes about three weeks to thoroughly dry. The skin should be like thin, crackly tissue paper. Store dried garlic bulbs in mesh bags or woven baskets in a dark, dry, cool location. If any bulbs begin to sprout, they must be used right away or they will rot.

A popular way to store garlic is by placing peeled cloves in olive oil in an airtight glass jar, and storing it in the refrigerator or an area that will prevent the mixture from getting above 45 degrees (dangerous bacteria from garlic will grow in oil that is warmer than 45 degrees).

As mentioned before, garlic has excellent medicinal properties. I recommend doing an in-depth study on this herb so you can be informed about the many benefits God combined in one plant! Loaded with nutrients, vitamins, minerals, many healing sulfur compounds, and more, this herb detoxifies the body, strengthens the immune system, is known to lower blood pressure, prevent ulcers, treat yeast infections, improve digestion, and is also helpful for treating colds and asthma. It acts as an overall tonic for the body.

Garlic is powerfully antiseptic and disinfectant. Taken internally, it prevents infection and keeps harmful bacteria from growing in the intestines and stomach. Some attest that taking a garlic supplement several times daily cleared up their acne and gave them a fresh complexion. Garlic supplements also help treat hay fever, sinus problems, and so much more! Topically, the distilled liquid of garlic effectively treats athlete's foot, boils, and other skin problems. So many ailments respond favorably to garlic, and I wouldn't have room to mention them all!

Of course, garlic has its problems too. If you take anticoagulants, avoid this herb. If you are susceptible to frequent indigestion, don't take large doses. And, oh yes, the odor…definitely not sweet! In fact, garlic has been called "the stinking rose" for centuries. After a meal including garlic, chew a sprig or two of fresh parsley or mint. If taking garlic supplements, look for the odorless type. It makes taking this herb a far more pleasant experience—for yourself and everybody around you!

But here I am, running out of space before I've even had a chance to discuss the simply wonderful culinary aspects of garlic! The fat little cloves are the main part to use, and are, of course, what we call "garlic." This part of the plant complements meat, poultry, seafood, and tomato-based dishes, enhancing and intensifying the natural flavor. The dried, powdered cloves are ever-so-good liberally rubbed over pork loin roast before baking! Simmer crushed cloves in your spaghetti and pizza sauces. Blend into butter or infuse in oil. Add to soups, mayonnaise, curries, and more! The juice of the cloves add zippy flavor to salad dressings and dips.

To make garlic powder, peel cloves, chop, and dry completely. Then grind and keep in an airtight container. You can add salt to make your own garlic salt seasoning mixture. Sprinkle this over just about any dish, from roast, to vegetables, to the traditional garlic bread!

Garlic does not lose its medicinal properties when cooked, but some suggest that the quality is slightly diminished when heated for a long period of time. To prevent this, add garlic during the last fifteen minutes of cooking, or avoid cooking over high heat.

The chive-like foliage of garlic has a deliciously mild garlic flavor. I recommend chopping them finely and adding fresh to garlic bread, baked potatoes, soups (just before serving), salads, pasta dishes, and wherever you would use chives or green onions. When too many leaves are harvested, the bulbs will be insignificant. If you develop a taste for garlic leaves, you might want to plant a bed specifically for the leaves!

Tips

Garlic is the gardener's friend, repelling most insect pests—especially aphids and Japanese beetles. Plant among your herbs and vegetables (except near beans and peas), and around your rosebushes. They also do well in borders.

A natural insect deterrent is made from crushed garlic cloves, cooking oil, water, and dish soap. Just soak a few fresh cloves in a teaspoon or two of oil for a few days, add a bit of soap, dilute with a gallon of water, and spray on infested plants.

MARJORAM

(Origanum majorana): Labiatae family, perennial. Zones 8–10.

Some claim that sweet marjoram and its cousin oregano are so similar that they don't need to be labeled separately. I am not of that opinion! Yes, the two are markedly similar (both being members of the genus *Origanum*), but they are also markedly different—which is why I am including an entry for each one!

First, I have an assignment for you. Go to your kitchen spice and seasoning rack. Take a taste of oregano, chewing it a little and letting it soften on your tongue so you can get the full flavor. Bold, pungent, and a little bitter, isn't it? Now take a drink of milk (to get rid of the taste), and try marjoram. Sweeter, wouldn't you say? A bit milder, but with a slight perfume taste that lingers. Now crush a bit of oregano between your fingers and smell it: sharp, fresh, and clean! Repeat with marjoram: gentle and more sweetly fragrant than oregano. Hmmm, it seems these cousins are uniquely individual—and it doesn't stop with scent and taste!

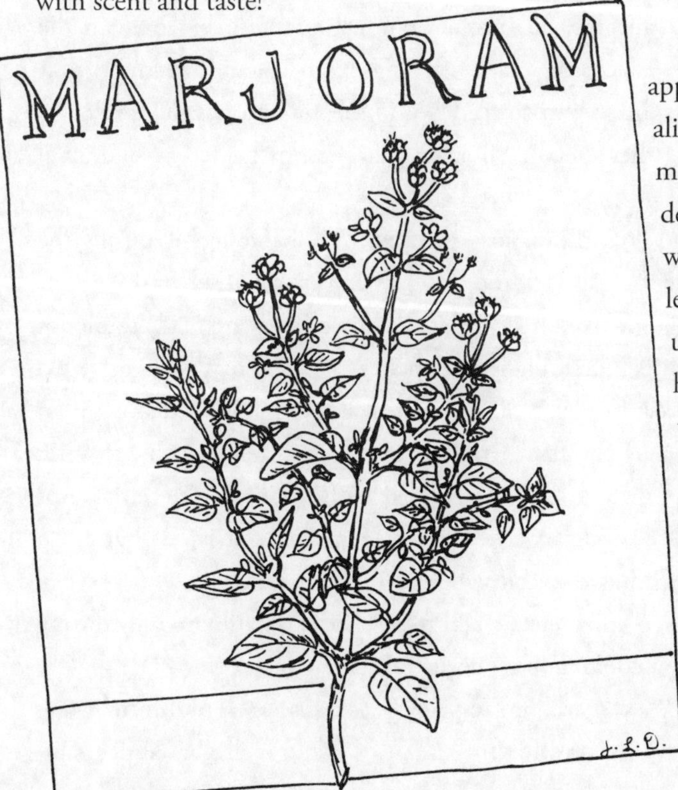

Although their appearance is strikingly alike, frost-tender marjoram is far more delicate than oregano, with softer, fuzzier leaves and a compact, upright growing habit—contrasting with oregano's dense, spreading growth. The leaves are a duller green than its cousin's light green ones, and not as firm. You will have to rub marjoram leaves to release their delicious perfume, since they meekly refrain from volunteering their fragrance! Both herbs bear small white to mauve flowers in midsummer that attract bees and butterflies.

Marjoram is easy to grow. You may sow seeds directly in the garden after the last spring frost, or start indoors about six weeks before the last frost date. Marjoram does best when propagated from cuttings or divisions, though, so perhaps a friend might let you take from their established plant. My simple solution is purchasing a plant from the local nursery!

Although relatively easy to grow, there are a few precautions: a sure way to destroy your plant is cold, wet soil and poor sun. Marjoram needs full sun and thrives in warm, dry, well-drained soil and light amounts of water. That is why I prefer to plant it in a container filled with a mixture of potting soil, perlite, and vermiculite. The container may be moved to catch the sun during the day, and brought into the garage or greenhouse at night if cool weather or frost is expected.

This lovely herb also does well in hanging baskets on the porch, or in a sunny windowsill indoors. It can grow all through winter indoors if cut back in the fall, but of course that weakens the plant. If you grow marjoram directly in your garden in mild climates, be sure to cut it down in the fall and possibly mulch to protect from winter weather. In cold climates, marjoram is treated as an annual or brought indoors.

Marjoram leaves and flowerheads may be used fresh, harvested all during the growing season. This herb dries well too, intensifying in flavor when dried. For drying, marjoram should be harvested just as the flowerheads are ready to bloom and the oil content is at its fullest. Hang in bunches in a dark, dry, well-ventilated area, or spread on a screen to dry. Rub from the stalk, crumble, and store in an airtight container. You may also freeze fresh, chopped marjoram in a bit of water in ice cube trays, or keep fresh leaves (sprinkled with water) in the refrigerator in a sealed container for about a week. Marjoram makes a delicious butter, so blend some into softened butter and it will keep nicely in your freezer for several months. When cooking, some prefer to add fresh or dried marjoram only during the last minute or two of cooking to retain its fullest flavor.

So far as medicinal uses, marjoram (especially as a tea) is helpful in relieving indigestion and in increasing sweating (to ease fevers), and it also has antioxidant properties. With a bit of honey, marjoram tea treats laryngitis and soothes overused vocal cords. It also helps relieve the symptoms of a bad cold. As a steam, it clears the sinuses. The oil of marjoram is sometimes combined with lavender essential oil and olive oil to rub on aches, pains, and muscle cramps. This works well for menstrual cramps. Poultices of the leaves help treat swelling. A diluted tea makes a good hair rinse, and you may add a few drops of the essential oil to shampoos to promote hair growth. As always, do your research before using. Some sources say that marjoram tea promotes menstruation and should be avoided by pregnant women; others declare that it is an effective treatment for morning sickness. Find a trustworthy source before using marjoram for medicinal purposes.

Marjoram is one of those herbs that lends itself delightfully to nearly any culinary use. It is considered a classic ingredient blended with dried thyme and sage. This seasoning mix makes its way into traditional stuffing, creating a pleasing, appetizing flavor most are familiar with. Marjoram is also popular added to sausage and meat loaf. The gentle taste makes it a good addition to mild foods such as poultry or egg-based dishes. Sprinkle some into your scrambled eggs toward the end of cooking—and enjoy a subtle boost of flavor! Add to vegetables the last thirty seconds of steaming, then serve as a special treat alongside baked chicken or turkey sandwiches (spread with marjoram butter!).

Marjoram is also excellent added to the batter of scones, biscuits, and dumplings. It blends well with butter, making a savory spread for fresh-baked bread, crackers, or sandwiches. The fresh or dried leaves may be added to soups (especially good in potato soup!) and stews for the last minute or two of cooking. Toss fresh leaves with your dinner salad or add a few to sandwich filling. Try some mixed in tuna fish and mayonnaise. Really, I do believe that marjoram goes well with just about everything! Why not add some to your meal this evening?

Tip

If you plant marjoram near the herb stinging nettle, it supposedly increases marjoram's essential oil content and promotes lush growth in both herbs. It's worth a try!

OREGANO

(Origanum vulgare): Labiatae family, perennial. Zones 5–9.

As we discussed before, oregano is often confused with its near relative marjoram, and is sometimes called "wild marjoram." While the herbs are similar in appearance, scent, and flavor, there is, as explained earlier, quite a difference!

Oregano tolerates cooler weather, is sturdy, dense, and has a spreading habit similar to (but not as invasive as) mint, and a flavor decidedly more robust, bold, and savory than marjoram. The scent is sharper and deliciously appetizing. Both herbs have tiny white or mauve flowers that form tight clusters at the top of the stems and bloom in midsummer. The leaves that cover the stems, and the tight flowerheads (picked just before they bloom), are the parts harvested for use.

You may propagate oregano by seed, cuttings, or root division, but I suggest purchasing plants from a nursery. That way you can skip the frustrations of trying to start a worthwhile oregano plant! There are quite a few variations of oregano, each with a slightly different taste. Go ahead and try a few! The key to getting a flavorful plant is to ask if you may taste a leaf before you buy.

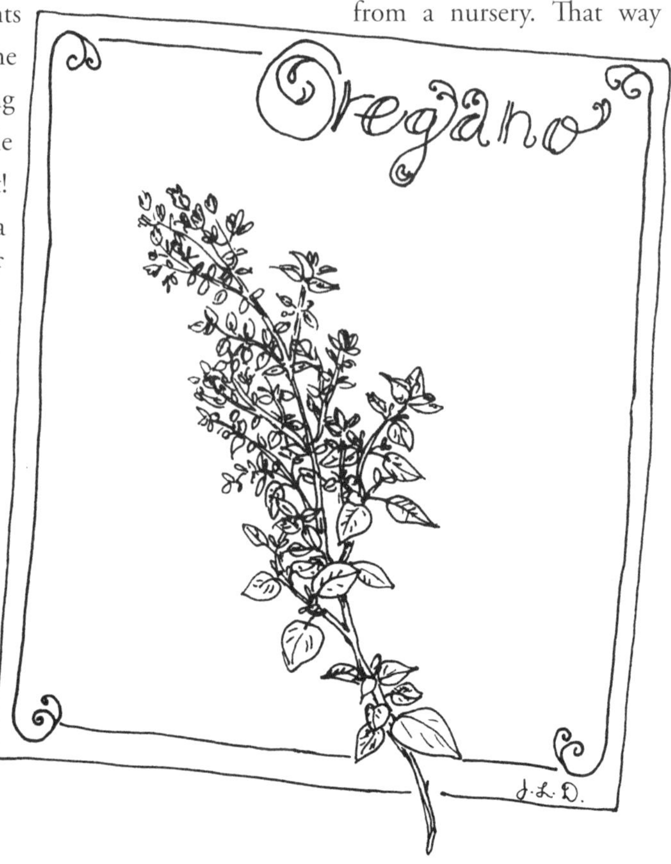

Plant well-rooted plants in slightly sandy,

well-drained soil and full sun. They also do well in containers in an average potting mix with a bit of perlite added. Don't overwater! This Mediterranean native likes hot, dry weather and can brave nearly any growing conditions—except soggy soil! Cut back oregano in the fall to promote healthy growth in the spring. If you live in a harsh climate, cover with mulch just after the first hard frost, and do not remove until after the last frost date.

To harvest (I suggest a thorough harvest twice during the growing season, and small harvests for fresh daily use whenever you feel like it!), snip stalks down near the base just before the flowerheads burst into bloom. Leave a few flowering stalks so that you won't miss out on the lovely, fragrant, bee-attracting blossoms! Hang bunches in a dark, dry, well-ventilated area and allow to dry until crumbly. Rub leaves and flowerheads from stalks and discard stalks.

Oregano does not lose its flavor when dried—in fact, it's actually enhanced by drying! You may also freeze finely chopped oregano in a bit of water in ice cube trays, or freeze or can in your spaghetti or pizza sauce.

Oregano is primarily a culinary herb, but it is considered a medicinal food that keeps winter illnesses at bay, supports the digestive tract, and relieves cramps. A tea may be taken to relieve menstrual cramps, irritability, and headaches. For topical use, oregano makes excellent infusions or bath sachets for a cleansing skin antiseptic, and an infused oil rub or compress may treat rheumatism and swelling joints. Essential oil may be diluted and applied to insect bites, or even an aching tooth! It also makes a good foot soak to treat athlete's foot. Many sources say that oregano's medicinal uses should be avoided by pregnant women.

In the kitchen, this may be one of the most frequently reached for herbs in the herb cabinet! Give a bit of dried oregano to a child, tell them to pop it into their mouth, and ask them what it tastes like. They'll probably close their eyes for a second, then shout, "Pizza!" Yes, oregano is what gives pizza sauce and other Italian favorites that flavor all their own. It can be found in Mexican salsa blends, many Greek dishes, and a myriad of American foods. Usually oregano is coupled with tomato-based dishes. Tomatoes bring out the flavor of the herb in a wonderfully tasty (and noticeable!) way. But tomatoes don't always have to be the base for oregano.

Toss spaghetti noodles in olive oil and sprinkle with fresh or dried oregano and grated Parmesan cheese. Accompany with basil in cheese and egg dishes. Add fresh leaves to dinner salads to serve alongside Italian dishes or soups. Blend into avocado dip. Use in place of marjoram for bolder flavor. Steam with vegetables such as zucchini. Add to bread crumbs for breading chicken and fish. Blend into cream cheese, cottage cheese, or softened butter. Sprinkle over garlic bread before baking. Include in bean dishes. Add dried, crushed leaves and those of dried parsley and basil for a tasty seasoning blend! And here's where oregano and marjoram are exactly the same: when cooking with them, the ideas are just about limitless!

Tips

This bee-attracting, pest-resistant herb is said to promote the growth of nearby plants.

Oregano does exceptionally well as a container herb—just be sure to have well-drained soil!

PARSLEY

"Curled Parsley" *(Petroselinum crispum):* Umbelliferae family, biennial. Zones 5-8.

Parsley is one of my most-loved herbs—both the bold and pretty common (or curled) parsley, and the flat-leaf Italian parsley (*P. crispum* var. *neapolitanum*).

What I like most about curled parsley is how graciously it lends itself to any container! I favor the crispy texture and mild flavor of this plant as well. It makes a pretty garden border and can be planted around the vegetable garden to keep parsley-loving animals (such as deer and rabbits) sidetracked from other plants. The flat leaves of Italian parsley are tender and deeply cut (resembling celery or lovage), and have stalks that can be used much like celery, if you let them grow large enough. I like the bright, cheery look of both varieties, their fresh flavor, invigorating aroma, and the wonderful health benefits that God wrapped into these tasty plants! In this entry, however, we will discuss common curled parsley.

Parsley is a low-maintenance herb that grows easily from seed (in cooler climates, start indoors six or seven weeks before the last spring frost). It thrives in rich, slightly acid, well-drained soil and full sun. As I said, curled parsley makes the perfect container plant, getting nearly two feet tall and rounding out to ten inches. You may keep a large pot of parsley on your kitchen counter (as long as there's lots of sun!) to harvest fresh parsley during the winter months. It makes a cheery reminder of summer, adding a bright, luscious green when so much outdoors is dull and colorless. The flavor, however, is best grown out of doors during the typical growing season.

In the spring of the second year, parsley sends up flowering stalks that produce tiny seeds. Save the seeds to start new plants. If you live in a cold climate, parsley will act as an annual. You may pot the plants to overwinter indoors, and then set them out again in the spring.

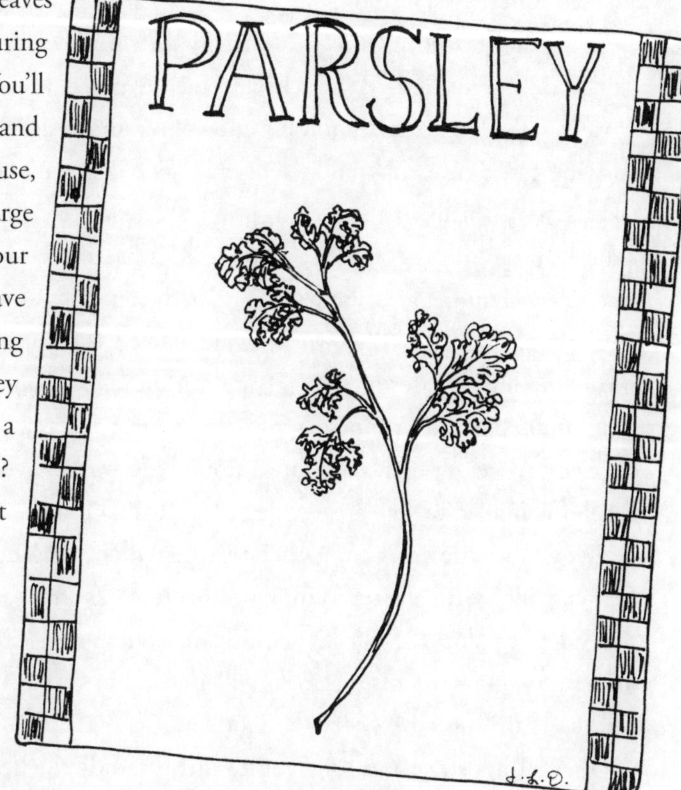

The firm, curly leaves can be harvested all during the growing season. You'll want to use them fresh and preserve for future use, so having several large clumps of parsley in your garden is a must! Have you ever tried sprinkling finely chopped parsley (fresh or dried) over a buttered baked potato? I think you'll agree that it's a delicious treat!

A good method for drying parsley (while retaining its vivid color) is as follows: Heat oven to 250 degrees. Arrange cut parsley on a baking sheet. Turn oven off and place baking sheet on the middle rack. Leave in the oven for about ten to fifteen minutes (until parsley is crumbly), turning several times. Cool completely and store in airtight containers away from light. You may also freeze finely chopped parsley in a bit of water in ice cube trays or freeze the whole leaves in airtight containers.

I found myself terribly undecided when it came to choosing which category to put parsley under—medicinal or culinary. It is wonderful for both. Of all the primarily culinary herbs termed "medicinal food," parsley takes the prize! From the bright green tops to the tiny seeds (technically called fruit and produced the second year), on down the stems, parsley is rich in vitamins, minerals, and is a strong antioxidant. According to Phyllis A. Blach and James F. Blach in their excellent book *Prescription for Nutritional Healing,* parsley contains more vitamin C than oranges by weight!

All parts of parsley are used for medicinal purposes except the flowers (the seeds are used for external purposes only). Like so many herbs, this one is also beneficial to the digestive tract. It helps treat urinary tract troubles, is helpful in eliminating kidney stones, and useful for relieving menstrual cramps. It also has wonderful properties that prevent the multiplication of tumor cells. Other helpful features are relieving gas, eliminating fluid retention, and lowering blood pressure. Some folks take parsley (usually in a tea) each spring as a general health tonic for the bladder, kidneys, liver, lungs, stomach, and thyroid. It has also been used to treat anemia. And so much more! Definitely *this* is an herb you will want to research further!

For topical uses, parsley works wonders too. The crushed leaves steeped in a small amount of water for topical application relieve pain and are antiseptic for skin troubles. Make a strong tea from the leaves, cool, and use to cleanse oily skin, close large pores, or reduce puffiness around the eyes. I have read that this infusion is helpful applied to sore areas suffered by nursing moms.

Remember the entry on garlic? I suggested chewing on a sprig of parsley to freshen your breath after consuming garlic. It works after eating chives and onions too! So don't skip the parsley garnish on your plate—it's there for more than looks! Eating a sprig after a meal will not only sweeten the breath, but it also stimulates the digestive system and kidneys.

There, I hope I've enthused you to further study the healthful benefits of this herb! Now let's see what it can do in the kitchen.

As far as flavor goes, both curled parsley and Italian bring to mind the fresh greenness of spring, but curled parsley is milder than Italian. That's where personal taste comes in, since they are interchangeable in cooking. Add fresh sprigs liberally to leaf salads, top soups (this is especially good in tortilla soup with sour cream!) and chowders, and use to perk up steamed vegetables.

Parsley is tasty with fish and seafood, complementing the flavors wonderfully. You can sprinkle crushed, dried parsley over beef steak too, for a nice flavor-booster. It's delicious in egg dishes—omelets, quiches, scrambled eggs, or sprinkled over fried eggs. And have you ever noticed that parsley blends well with potatoes in any form? Try adding some to your next potato salad—it's yummy!

You may add parsley to white sauces, tomato dishes, or boil with turnips. Steam with peas and carrots, and then toss in butter! The flavor of parsley blends well with garlic, making it a mouthwatering combination, mixed with butter or olive oil, to spread over French bread and toast to a crusty brown. Mix dried parsley with dried chervil, chives, and tarragon—the well-known *fines herbes* blend. And I've read that in Morocco cooks combine Italian parsley with coriander in many of their dishes. Give it a try if you enjoy variety!

Fresh parsley sprigs stand alone as a unique side dish when deep-fried. You may also use the fresh sprigs in stir-fries with mushrooms, onions, and garlic. Fresh sprigs of parsley are a lovely, cheery garnish to any meal.

Now, after discussing all of that, let's step outside on the back deck. I suppose you aren't surprised to see brimming pots of parsley! Oh, yes—that's my herb garden over there with many brilliant mounds as a border. Pretty, isn't it? And here, you may take these extra parsley starts home, if you'd like—they'll add delightfully to your garden!

Tips

Plant parsley among your roses and tomatoes—it really seems to help them thrive!

Even if you don't want the seeds, let parsley flower the second year. The honeybees will thank you!

SAGE

(Salvia officinalis): Labiatae family, perennial. Zones 4–8.

Common sage stands on its own for flavor. Once you've tasted it, you really can't liken it to any other taste. Some call it bitter, others pungent, and still others take a bite, close their eyes, and simply say, "Ummm! Delicious!"

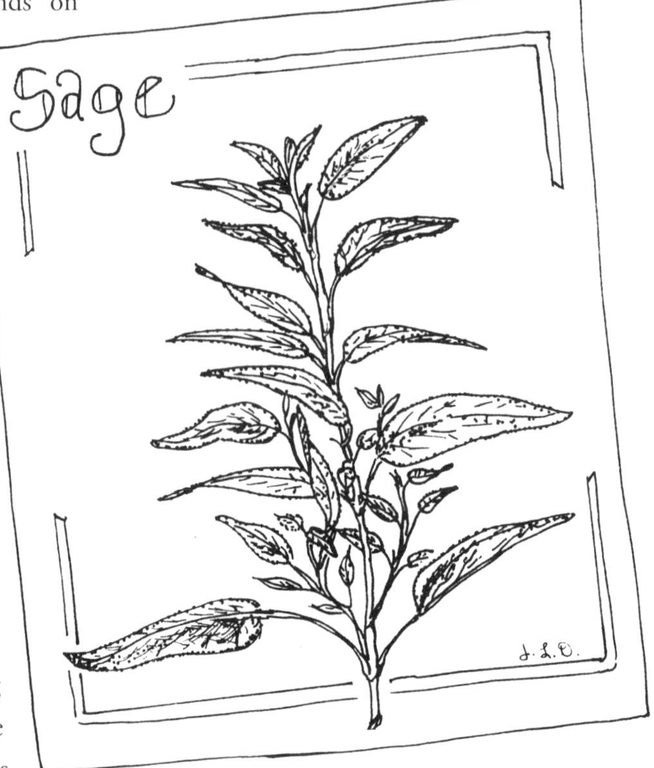

For most of us, the flavor holds pleasant memories of the stuffing that goes so well with our Thanksgiving turkey or alongside poultry. Anyone who has read Laura Ingalls Wilder's *Little House on the Prairie* books might remember the argument she and her sister Mary had in *By the Shores of Silver Lake.* With the larder nearly empty and game scarce, Pa was out hunting a goose for Thanksgiving dinner. Laura—who disliked the flavor of sage—wanted Ma to season the stuffing with onion. Mary insisted on sage. In the end Pa came home without a goose. Years later Laura wrote, "I remember saying in a meek voice to sister Mary, 'I wish I had let you have the sage.'"[1] But sage is like that—a flavor either loved, barely tolerated, or despised. Judging from the popularity of this herb in the culinary realm, however, the majority of people side with Mary!

1 *"Laura and Mary Quarrel at Thanksgiving," page 302,* Little House in the Ozarks: The Rediscovered Writings of Laura Ingalls Wilder, *edited by Stephen W. Hains, Tennessee. Thomas Nelson Publishers. 1991.*

Sage is more than a tasty seasoning. The two-foot-tall rounded shrub is an attractive addition to the herb garden—in the ground or gracing a container. Its silvery-green, sandpapery, pointed leaves burst with volatile oils and tannins, and are highly aromatic—a scent somewhat like lemon with a touch of camphor. In late summer, edible purple, two-lipped flowers cover the stalks with a burst of exquisite color, attracting honeybees, hummingbirds, and butterflies. Sage is worth its space in the garden even if you only grow it for the gorgeous display of flowers! But after discovering its many culinary and medicinal uses, I imagine most folks will be drawn to experiment with this popular plant.

Sage is a hardy perennial and fairly easy to grow. You may purchase seeds and start indoors or direct-sow, but it takes at least two years to get a bush of worthwhile size. I prefer purchasing a well-rooted plant, then a year or two later propagating from this plant by cuttings, layering, or root division. Root division is my first choice, layering a close second. Sage grows to about two feet tall and wide, so space accordingly. Basic needs are simple: well-drained soil, full sun, wind protection, and light watering. Cut plants back in the fall or spring, and be sure to cover with mulch in the fall if you live in harsh climates. Sage is drought-tolerant, doesn't mind cool weather, loves sunshine, and resists pests and diseases. A sure way to destroy your plant, though, is to let the soil get soggy. Sage can't stand wet feet.

To harvest the leaves, do so just before the flowers bloom. Hang bunches in a dry, dark, well-ventilated area, allowing to dry until crumbly. Sage that isn't thoroughly dry will mold. Once dry, remove from stalks and crumble the leaves into airtight containers. Don't worry if the dried leaves look fuzzy—since sage leaves are covered with downy little hairs, dried sage will appear that way. You may also freeze fresh sage in the simple ice-cube-tray method, or blend into butter and freeze.

Sage is more than just a tasty seasoning and attractive sight. It has been counted among the most valued medicinal herbs for centuries, making it fall under the category of "medicinal food" when used in cooking. Sage is loaded with nutrients and vitamins, plus it has astringent and tonic properties. It is known to be of special benefit for treating ailments of the throat and mouth—an infusion of the leaves making an excellent antiseptic gargle or mouthwash. It even whitens the teeth! Sage also stimulates the digestive tract and central nervous system, is beneficial for women's health (it is said to be good for treating estrogen deficiency in menopause and after a hysterectomy), promotes hair growth and revitalizes dark hair when used as a topical rinse, is helpful when added to skin creams, eases joint pain when applied topically, and much more!

As with all medicinal herbs, sage has some cautions. Used for culinary purposes, it is considered healthful and harmless. But internal medical uses (such as medicinal-strength teas, etc.) may interfere with the absorption of iron and other minerals, and decrease milk supply in nursing mothers. (Also, the flavor comes through in the milk, and most babies agree with Laura—not Mary—about the flavor!) It has also been cautioned that sage (except in small amounts in cooking) should not be used by those who have seizures, or by pregnant women. So, as always, before using for medicinal purposes (internal or topical), *do your research!*

But let's get back to the main point of this entry: culinary uses of this delightful herb! Because of its strong flavor, sage can be used alone to season poultry, fish, beef, and pork. It is a common ingredient in sausage and goes especially well with fatty or oily foods, assisting the digestion. Since sage is a very strong-tasting herb, many prefer blending it with other herbs, such as thyme and marjoram, or garlic, basil, and tarragon, or with ground black pepper. That's my favorite way, but suit your taste! Add to pea soup, bean dishes, chowders, and stews. Mix a pinch in dumpling batter. Stir into cream sauces for a special touch.

Sage also goes well with tomatoes, eggs, cheese (it makes a yummy spread mixed with cream cheese or sprinkled over sharp cheddar), butter, biscuits, and breads. And of course it is exceptional (according to some people!) in poultry stuffing!

Sage may be used fresh or dried, and the flowers either candied for use as pretty edible garnishes or tossed fresh in salads. The candied leaves make lovely and helpful after-dinner "mints" (remember, sage is in the mint family!), easing indigestion and sweetening the breath.

Tips

For a lovely effect, plant rosemary and sage side by side in borders or containers. More than just lovely, they encourage growth in each other as well.

Sage repels the cabbage butterfly, making it the perfect herb to grow among your cabbage rows.

SAVORY

(Winter savory, *Satureja montana;* Summer savory, *S. hortensis):* Labiatae family, Winter savory, perennial; summer savory, annual. Zones 5–9.

Remember how cilantro and coriander are like two herbs in one plant? Well, winter savory and its cousin summer savory are like one culinary herb in two different plants! Since both types of savory are used in the same way, choosing which to add to your herb garden is up to you. Winter savory is considered just a bit bolder in taste, while the summer variety is sweeter, like thyme, with a hint of peppery mint. Each contains the same sharp, spicy flavor reminiscent of black pepper, only milder and more, well, *savory*! However, despite the slight differences in taste, savories are commonly used interchangeably. I suppose that works! But for myself, growing both varieties and using according to taste is the best choice!

In the garden, savories add an artistic touch. They're both quite pretty in different ways! The hardy winter variety grows to about fifteen inches tall, twelve inches around, and with a strong root system. It is a stiff, compact shrub with narrow, dark green leaves. Grown in well-drained potting soil with a bit of perlite added, this makes a compact potted herb that can easily be moved to catch the sun, or kept indoors during harsh winters. If you live in a climate where the winter temperatures do

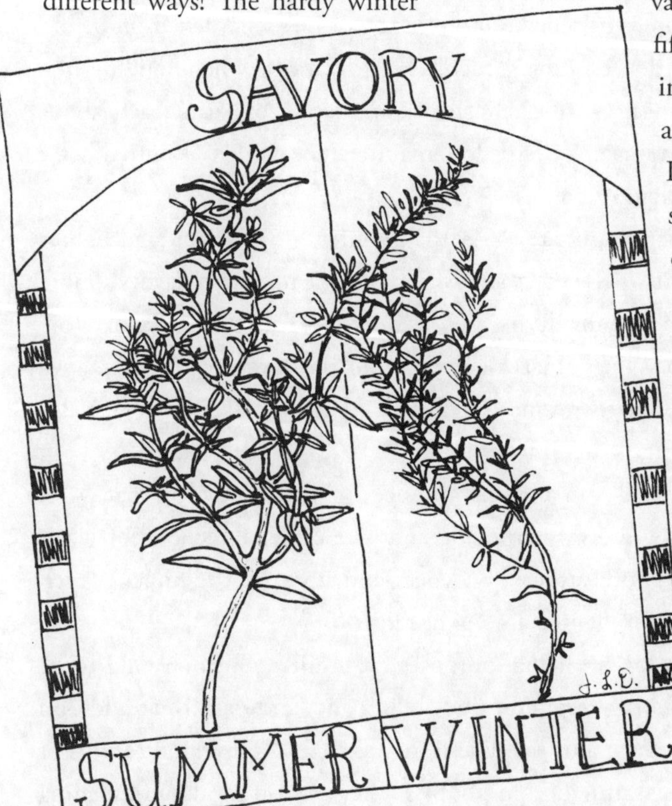

not drop below 10 degrees, you may grow winter savory directly in your garden and simply cut back in the fall and mulch well after the first hard frost. In temperate climates, winter savory is a hardy evergreen.

In late summer, a lovely mist of white or lavender flowers come into bloom. Harvest leaves just as this is happening, using fresh or hanging in bunches to dry in a dark, dry, well-ventilated area or on a baking sheet at 110 degrees until crumbly. Discard stems and store leaves in an airtight container. You may propagate winter savory by seed, but root divisions, or tip cuttings from new growth, are a better choice. Perhaps a friend will let you take from their established plant! Winter savory does well for about three years, and then becomes woody and straggly and should be replaced.

Summer savory is far more delicate and cannot endure frost or cold soil. It grows easily from seed, whether directly in the garden or as a potted plant. Start seeds at least six weeks before the last spring frost, and be careful when planting in the garden—seedlings are very delicate and must be properly hardened-off before permanent summer residence in the garden! Use special care when handling the delicate roots of seedlings. Once established, summer savory can reach about eighteen inches tall, and makes a pretty, low-maintenance garden or potted herb. It requires more water than its cousin.

The leaves of summer savory are softer than winter, a bit longer, and lighter green with a bronze tint. It has erect stems (in contrast to winter savory's more trailing habit), and is better for drying because it retains its strong flavor more than dried winter savory does. Harvest just before the lovely white or mauve flowers begin to bloom in late summer. Near the end of the season, you may also uproot the entire plant and hang it to dry.

Both savories require full sun and well-drained, slightly sandy soil that won't become soggy. The leaves are very aromatic and give off a pungent scent when crushed. The flowers of both attract honeybees and improve the honey, which explains why they are often planted among beehives.

The uses of savories for medicinal purposes are similar. Both are said to be highly beneficial for treating respiratory troubles, colic, and gas. Their addition to foods (especially legumes) aids the digestion. Taken as topical applications or internally, savories are healthful for skin troubles. They are also good for freshening the breath and cleansing the digestive system. Fresh, crushed leaves applied to a bee sting bring immediate relief.

But what about their culinary attractions? The peculiar, hot, keenly sharp taste is delicious cooked in lentil, pea, or bean soups—the traditional use for this herb. In fact, in Germany it is called *bohnenkraut*, meaning "bean herb." But don't limit savory to bean dishes. Try it in white sauces and gravies. Add to flour, cornmeal, or bread crumbs with lemon basil to coat butter-dipped fish or chicken before frying—it's good! Add to sauces for seafood. Sprinkle fresh winter savory in slow-cooking stew—it will intensify the flavor. Savory also makes a tasty fresh vegetable marinade when added to lemon juice and vinegar, with a few garlic cloves and a touch of honey. Or add when sautéing mushrooms in butter—you can't beat the absolutely delicious combination!

The fresh leaves of both savories are nice for perking up dinner salads, and why not try some fresh or dried savory in poultry stuffing? Some favor it above the usual sage seasoning (probably Laura Ingalls Wilder would have preferred it!). It is also delicious when added, fresh and finely chopped, to biscuit batter or bread dough. Or simply use finely crushed dried savory in place of ground black pepper at the dinner table.

The essential oil is sometimes used as a flavoring in salami and other foods, but be sure to follow a tried-and-true recipe for that—the oil is exceedingly strong.

Tips

Plant savory near onions and green beans—it supposedly promotes growth in all. Besides that, all three make a tasty combination sautéed together!

Indoor pots of summer savory benefit from having their leaves misted.

THYME

(Garden thyme, *Thymus vulgaris;* Lemon thyme, *T. x citriodorus):* Labiatae family, perennial. Zones 5–9.

"Culinary or medicinal—what section should I put thyme in?" The question came to me as I sat down to write about this tremendously beneficial herb (a pot of which beautifies the sunny windowsill by my desk). The leaves contain vitamin A, nicacin, potassium, calcium, and iron, making it a health food worth cooking and doctoring with! But despite its excellency in the medicinal field, I chose to focus on the culinary attraction of this flavorful herb.

In the mint family, thyme (pronounced "tīm" or "thīm") is another herb with numerous varieties. Garden thyme and lemon thyme (a hybrid cross) are most commonly used in cooking, so we'll discuss these two tasty types!

All thyme varieties are perennials. You may propagate from seed, cuttings, or (with garden thyme) root division. For a head start, I suggest purchasing a well-rooted plant at the nursery, and then in a year or two propagating from this plant by cuttings or (again, for garden thyme) root division. After four or five years, your first plant will probably need to be replaced to insure production quality.

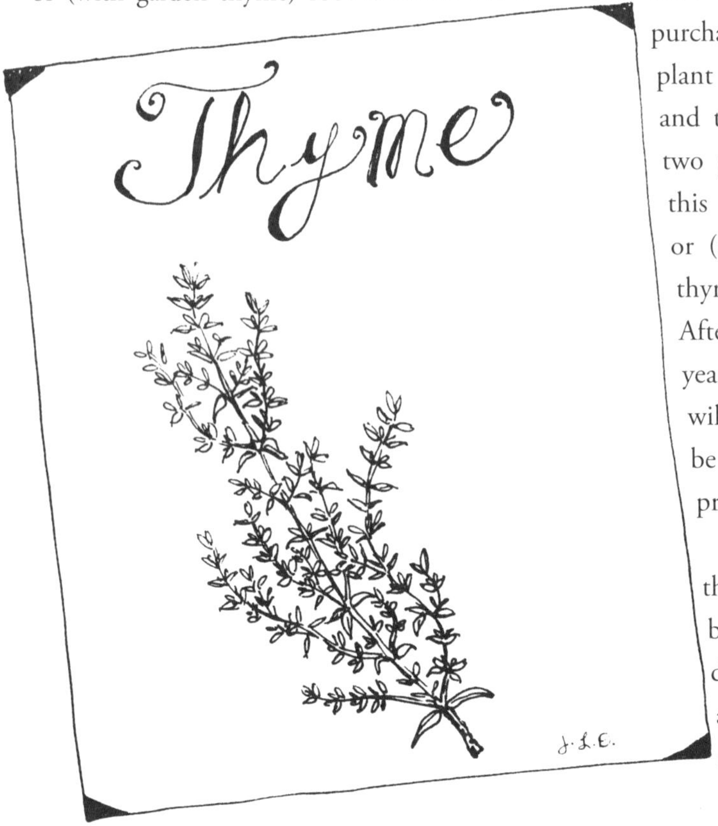

The leaves of thyme are tiny—but pungent—and densely cover the abundant slender stalks. Rub a leaf between your fingers, releasing the oils and filling the air with a fresh, heady aroma that is delicious—even more so in the lemon variety! Watch for a frosty mantle of color in early summer when bee-attracting clusters of tiny white, purple, or pink flowers cover the plants. The leaves of garden thyme have a gray-green tint, covering the erect, bushy, twelve-inch-tall plant. Lemon thyme has just a bit larger leaves of a greener hue, reaches only about six inches in height, and has an attractive spreading habit that makes it drape charmingly over the edges of containers, or trail picturesquely down hillsides or over rocks in a rock garden. Both types of thyme thrive in full sun and light, well-drained, dry soil. In fact, their flavor is far stronger if grown in hot, dry climates. Because of its far-reaching root system, thyme could quickly invade the surrounding plants. You can avoid this by planting each thyme in its own container.

Harvest leafy branches just before they flower. To dry, hang bunches in a dark, dry, well-ventilated place until fully dried. Remove from stalks, but don't crush the leaves until you're cooking with them (the leaves retain their oils better if stored whole). Unlike some herbs, thyme retains its strong flavor even after it's dried. Store in an airtight container. You may also freeze whole sprigs of thyme in sealed containers, or finely chopped fresh thyme in a bit of water in ice cube trays, and yes! this herb is delightful blended into butter too, so go ahead and freeze some.

Thyme, as we mentioned, has some very beneficial uses in the medicinal realm. It supports the immune system, fights coughs and colds, and treats respiratory troubles. This is one of my favorite herbs to use in infused honey or syrups to treat sore throats and coughs, and it also makes healing ointments and balms for topical purposes. As a nutritious tea, it treats digestive troubles. Sore muscles are gently eased when an infusion of thyme is added to the bath. Infusions also help in treating skin troubles and improving skin texture. Lemon thyme is especially helpful for children's health, because they tend to enjoy the delicious, sweet taste, while it calms upset stomachs, eases sore throats, and supports immune and digestive health. A simple cough syrup is made from an infusion of thyme leaves, strained and blended into honey. Take by the tablespoon for adults and teaspoon for children several times a day. Refrigerate for four to five days.

In the kitchen, thyme is wonderful! Fresh or dried, the leaves of either garden or lemon thyme (depending on your preference in taste) are the perfect accompaniment to soups, stews, vegetable dishes, fish, lamb, poultry, omelets, and so much more! Yes, it even makes a delightfully different seasoning for poultry stuffing. Thyme is what lends that "certain" flavor (noticeably tasty!) to clam and fish chowders. Its warm, unique taste stands up to long periods of cooking and blends especially well with garlic, olives, and tomatoes, making it a common ingredient in Italian sauces and spice mixes. For a perfect accompaniment to a tossed salad, split a loaf of French bread, drizzle with olive oil, sprinkle liberally with fresh or dried thyme leaves, top with grated Parmesan cheese, and toast until deliciously crusty. Yum! You may also make your own savory herb blend by mixing dried thyme with other dried herbs, such as parsley, sage, and oregano. Store in a shaker and keep near your stove to conveniently season foods. Oh, and did I mention that lemon thyme can make a refreshing, nourishing, super-tasty tea? Try it steeped with a few peppermint leaves (and a bit of honey) for a relaxing moment on the porch swing with a good book!

Tips

Thyme repels cabbage maggots and moths.

Mother-of-thyme *(T. serpyllum)* makes a good ground cover among fruit trees, since the flowers strongly attract bees to pollinate your trees!

OTHER CULINARY HERBS TO LEARN MORE ABOUT

***Sunflower** (Helianthus annuus)*

Comes in varieties from two to twelve feet tall, or taller! Sturdy stalks with large, heart-shaped leaves and bright yellow flowers having dark brown centers crammed with seeds—and seeds are the part used.

Vitamin and mineral rich, the seeds (and oil made from the seeds) combine nutritious with delicious! Boasting a mild, nutty taste, these go well in baked goods, sprinkled over salads, standing alone as a tasty snack, and so much more. Don't forget that birds especially love sunflower seeds. Why not plant a few sunflowers just for them?

***Lemon Verbena** (Aloysia triphylla)*

Graceful perennial shrub in zones 7–8; does well in the greenhouse. Long, pointed citral-rich leaves of a soft pale green. Purple flowers bloom in midsummer.

The deliciously sweet-scented leaves burst with lemon aroma and flavor. Perfect in tea, or chopped and added to stuffing, poultry, and fish. Toss fresh in salads. Use in jams and jellies. Excellent! Has good medicinal qualities as well.

***Watercress** (Nasturtium officinale)*

Bright green, glossy, low-growing plant with hollow stems. White blossoms from midsummer.

Bursting with vitamins, calcium, and iron. Harvest as soon as leaves are large enough. It's peppery-hot, refreshingly tangy, and tasty in soups, salads, steamed like kale, and more. The seeds produce delicious, crunchy, highly nutritious sprouts that are wonderful on whole wheat bread spread with butter! Contains medicinal value.

Almighty

Sun, moon, and stars, the mighty, rolling sea—
His great voice spoke, and it all came to be!
He who has brought such lofty works to being,
Has also made each minute, little thing.
Praise to the Lord, who formed this lovely world;
From mountain height, to tender herb unfurled.
Praise to the Lord, who, making, never spared
His best for us for whom earth was prepared.
–J.L.D.

All things were made by him (John 1:3).

Top Fifteen Medicinal Herbs

And God said, Behold, I have given you every herb bearing seed, which is upon the face of all the earth, and every tree, in the which is the fruit of a tree yielding seed; to you it shall be for meat (Genesis 1:29).

Medicinal herbs are those that have strong healing properties. For centuries they have been used to treat and prevent illnesses and disorders. Used with caution and wisdom, medicinal herbs offer a safe and natural remedy for many of the body's ailments.

God expects us to cultivate practical as well as spiritual wisdom. Typically, when we first begin working with herbs as medicine, we are careful to use our God-given practical wisdom. We do our research, obey cautions, and precisely measure out doses. While a small amount of leeway is often safe when working with herbs, a healthy respect for the powerful components God created in them is a good thing!

Unfortunately, I've noticed that frequent use of herbs tends to make us less cautious than we should be. As we grow familiar with making our own medicine, we lose some of that wise caution so necessary for safe use of medicinal herbs. Don't let this happen! Research and continue to read widely, even about herbs you are familiar with.

Label and date all herbal preparations. It may be helpful to write a list of medicinal herbs you use frequently, and note any cautions, which parts are for what, and which parts are not for ingestion. This quick-reference guide not only saves time, but also maintains safety. Be sure to put highlighted cautions beside dangers that may apply to you or your family, such as herbs not to be used during pregnancy, lactation, by children, by those with heart problems, by those on certain medications, etc. This isn't an overreaction—it may protect a life! Post the list as a handy reference on the inside of the cabinet door where you store medicinal herbs.

The following pages profile fifteen of my favorite healing and supportive medicinal herbs. And the profiles are simply that: basic overviews intended to spark your interest and inspire further research. Do you suffer from colon troubles, frequent colds, skin rashes, stress, muscle aches, respiratory troubles, or other common problems? Perhaps one of the fifteen favorite medicinal herbs will be your key to relief!

Remember, the author of this book does not profess to be an expert or professional. The following profiles are not intended to take the place of professional medical advice from your doctor or qualified persons. Always consult your physician with medical questions, and research carefully before using herbs for medicinal purposes.

Joy is distinctly a Christian word. It is the reverse of happiness. Happiness is the result of what happens of an agreeable sort. Joy has its springs deep down inside. Only Jesus gives that joy. –S.D. Gordon

ALOE VERA

(Aloe barbadensis): Liliaceae family, perennial. Zone 3.

It isn't hard for me to choose a favorite medicinal/skin care herb! Safe and effective for so many purposes, aloe vera comes out on top. I call it the "Miracle Plant."

As alluded to in chapter one, this herb came as an answer to prayer concerning inflamed skin troubles. And that isn't all! Through the years it has helped in promoting overall health. I'll write more about that in a moment, but first let me give a little information on the herb itself.

A member of the lily family but strongly resembling a cactus, aloe needs dry, sandy soil, hot weather, and filtered sun exposure. It is a succulent with tender, fleshy leaves that seal up after you pinch off a piece. Native to East Africa, aloe also thrives in countries like Spain. In the United States it does especially well in parts of California and Texas, where it is grown commercially. If you live in a cooler climate, aloe makes a nice houseplant that thrives on neglect, filtered sun, and very little water! In fact, it is best to water aloe only once a month. Give it a thorough (but not sopping wet) watering, then leave it alone for another month! Choose a potting mix formulated for cacti/succulents.

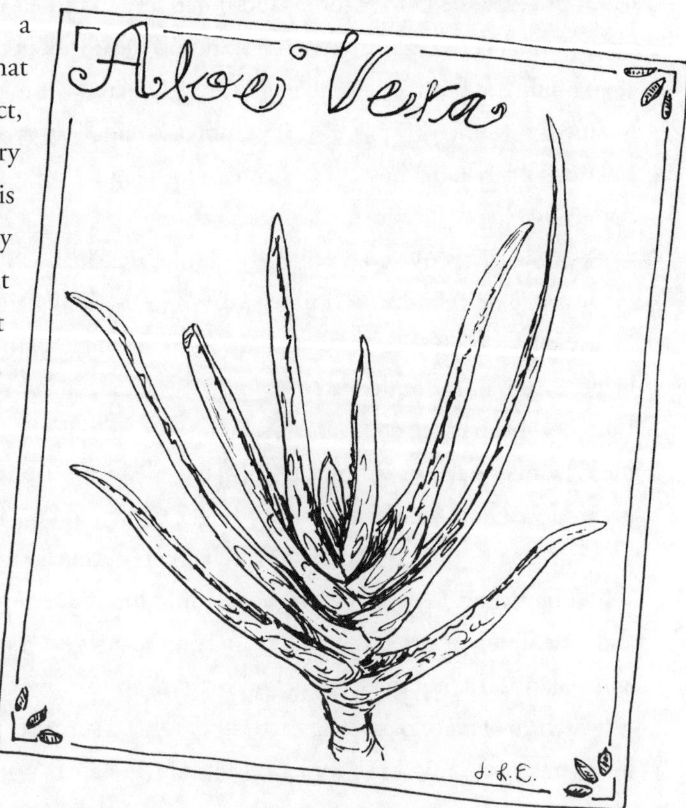

Aloe vera leaves grow in a rosette from the base. Harvest only the outer leaves. You can pinch off little bits at a time as needed, or gently remove a whole leaf, but don't harvest too many or the plant will die. The simplest way to propagate is by rooting the suckers that form around the base. It takes about three years before aloe produces flowering stalks of orange or red blooms.

Aloe's bright, spring-green color adds a cheerful glow to kitchen windowsills and serves as a handy "first-aid kit." The clear, nutrient-rich gel in the thorn-edged leaves acts as a natural astringent, antiseptic, and speeds up the healing process. It is perfect for soothing and healing rashes, cuts, and burns—especially sunburns. Snip off the end of an aloe spear (as the leaves are called), squeeze out the gel on the affected area, and find immediate relief! It also helps prevent scarring.

But aloe gel isn't for topical uses alone. Drinking a bit of the slightly bitter juice works wonders to promote regularity and colon health, acts as a soothing remedy for digestive tract irritations, is a mild nerve sedative, lowers cholesterol, improves circulation in the lower extremities, soothes and heals stomach and esophagus irritation, acts as a kidney tonic, and much, much more! Always do your research before using. Although proven to be safe and healthful, herbal guides caution that aloe should not be taken internally during pregnancy (it may trigger contractions), by nursing women (it passes through breast milk), or by those with rare allergic reactions or irritable bowel syndrome. Don't ingest on a regular basis for longer than two weeks, since it may work too strongly as a laxative.

So, now that we've covered the basics, let me share what sparked my personal interest in aloe vera nearly thirteen years ago. Suffering from inflamed blemishes on my face, I tried everything I could think of to clear up the problem. Nothing helped, from home remedies to expensive visits at the dermatologist. That is, until I discovered that the soothing, healing effect of aloe gel isn't merely for burned fingers, small cuts, or sunburns—it's also effective on blemishes and rashes! My discovery came when I burned my finger while baking. I quickly snipped off a piece of aloe to put on the burn. It felt so good that I suddenly wondered what would happen if I tried aloe on the burning inflammation on my face. I tried it, and it definitely relieved the hot feeling! So the next day I purchased several plants and began spreading the fresh gel on my face at least five times a day, using a new half-inch-long piece of the leaf each time. What a surprise! After years of searching for an answer to my skin problem, I found true relief. Within a week there was a noticeable improvement on my face. After several months of this application, my condition was so well under control that I was no longer embarrassed to go out in public. After a year of daily use, the problem I had suffered with for nearly eight years was completely gone, never to return!

But by that time I had learned that frequent use of aloe on the skin does more than simply *clear up* skin problems; it moistens and nourishes the skin, keeps it youthful, protects against future problems, and feels so refreshing! However, I didn't have room to start an aloe vera farm, and using the gel daily takes a lot of aloe! That's when I began testing bottled aloe vera gel products on the market. Some worked great but were too costly. Some had harmful or irritating preservatives. But through trial and error, it has been fun to find those products that are *almost* as good as fresh-picked aloe!

Recent years have brought about discoveries in preserving aloe, but few are adaptable to home-preserving without sacrificing quality. You can make a homemade gel by carefully peeling off the skin and blending the gel with vitamin C powder (500 units per cup of gel). This mixture lasts for about two weeks in the refrigerator, but it is rather inconvenient to make and uses up a lot of aloe! Unless you have quite a few plants, it really isn't worth it. I suggest purchasing bottled aloe vera gel for uses that exceed small cuts and burns. Look for products of full-strength gel labeled for internal use (this works for both internal and external purposes). Be sure it has been preserved using the cold-pressed method, since it allows aloe vera to retain its natural polysaccharide-rich properties. Aloe vera gel from Aloe Farms® (available through Nature's Warehouse, see page 225) is one of my favorite bottled aloe products. It's great for internal use (I mix ¼ cup with cranberry juice), but also luxuriant when added to shampoos, creams, and lotions. I even like to smooth it on my skin full-strength for a quick refresher. Wonderful!

Aloe vera gel makes a wonderful base for essential oils such as tea tree oil or lavender oil. It helps the oils spread on evenly and penetrate the surface quicker to work their healing wonders.

If you have an aloe vera plant that has grown shaggy, withered, and dusty, hopefully this entry will encourage you to give it a bit of attention and start putting it to use!

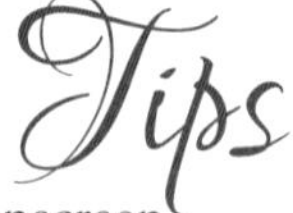

The aloin in aloe acts as a mild sunscreen.

Kathy Keville, in her book *Herbs: An Illustrated Encyclopedia*, notes that aloe's pH is about 4.3—perfect for skin, since its pH is between 4 and 6!

Aloe is virtually pest free, but once in a while mealybugs will infest a plant. Gently wipe infested leaves with a cotton ball soaked in rubbing alcohol. Wash treated leaves before using.

CALENDULA

(Calendula officinalis): Compositae family, annual, sometimes biennial.

Calendula, a beautiful herb with radiant golden yellow to orange flowers, shines in the medicinal herb garden. Adding it to the flower garden is a lovely idea too. And it shouldn't be kept out of the culinary garden either! Also called "pot marigold" (which doesn't allude to the herb being grown in pots, but rather to its tasty, colorful addition to the soup pot), calendula is sometimes confused with true marigolds *(Tagetes genus),* which are not herbs. Don't get them mixed up, since the two are not interchangeable!

Calendula is a hardy annual that grows almost anywhere. It is propagated from seeds sown directly into roughed-up garden soil in the fall or early spring. If sown in the fall, expect blooms sometime around April (or, in climates like mine, June!). Once the soil has warmed (to about 55 degrees), it takes at least two weeks for seeds to sprout. Growing in clumps, calendula is not spread by roots or runners. However, it doesn't self-seed very well either. You will want to help it out by harvesting the dry seeds in the fall and scattering them in the soil. Once established, calendula likes light water, full sun, and nearly any type of soil that isn't soggy.

Calendula actually blooms in a more prolific way when the weather is cool and the flowers are picked frequently—which is wonderful, because the flowers are the part you want to harvest all through the growing season! The large, lovely blossoms (made up of many small petal rays) open bright and early in the morning, and close just as evening comes. They are supported by sturdy, deep green 10- to 24-inch-tall stalks, and have long, oblong, tender green leaves and a long taproot.

Calendula flowers offer a wide sphere of usefulness. They make sturdy, beautiful cut flowers, are delightful in the flower garden, and yet useful for many purposes, from making a creamy yellow dye to adding a lovely hue and healthful boost to soups, stews, and sauces, and acting as a healing ingredient in salves and creams. The tasty, salty-sweet petals (pulled loose, one by one, from the head), and sometimes the young leaves (though slightly acrid tasting), are used as a bright, flavorful addition to leaf salads. Dried calendula flowers make a golden food coloring for tea, soup, rice, stew, and even frosting. They can be used as a substitute for true saffron for adding color and flair.

This lovely herb's medicinal and body care uses far exceed any other of its attractions. It is known to kill bacteria and fungi, and is used as a remedy against candida. It is gentle enough to be applied (in a weak infusion in water) to thrush in infants' mouths. Adults may use a stronger infusion as a mouthwash to treat toothache.

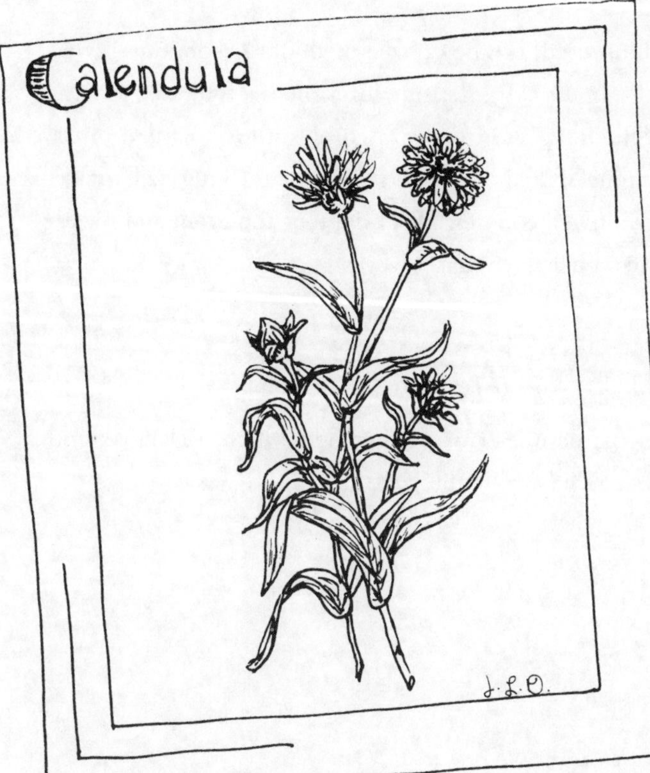

Gentle and soothing, calendula is a popular ingredient in baby oils, creams, soaps, and salves. The dried and ground petals make a good baby powder when mixed with cornstarch. Due to its nonirritating, healing properties, calendula (added to gentle creams or aloe vera gel) is good for treating diaper rash and other skin troubles common to infants and small children. For older children and adults, it makes an excellent hair rinse for light hair, is beneficial for sensitive skin, soothes mild burns and sunburn, decreases inflammation of sprains, varicose veins, and other swellings, and helps treat most rashes. One especially wonderful use is a strong infusion made from the flower petals in water, cooled, and splashed over skin eruptions of chicken pox or measles, relieving discomfort and speeding up the healing process. This can also be used to treat acne.

I have not experimented with the internal uses of calendula, but researching the subject indicates it is good for many ailments. It is said to help regulate the menstrual cycle, lower fever, and treat tonsillitis by promoting drainage of swollen lymph glands. It also has helpful uses in therapy for uterine and breast cancer. I strongly recommend investing in a concise guide to using calendula internally before venturing to do so.

Calendula flowers (fresh or dried) can be utilized in all of the common herbal preparations, treating many ailments. Try a strong infusion as a foot soak to treat skin ailments of the feet. Smooth a bit of the infused oil on for a natural insect repellent. Or simply pluck some of the fresh flowers (keeping the long stalk intact) and place in a vase on your kitchen counter. This brightens the room and makes you feel more cheery. I think you'll agree that it works!

Tip

Plant calendula around the perimeter of your gardens (herb, vegetable, and flower). It is said to sidetrack aphids, whiteflies, and thrips.

CHAMOMILE

(Matricaria recutita): Compositae family, annual.

Chamomile (sometimes spelled camomile) is one of the most well-known and often-used medicinal herbs. It makes itself useful in so many ways—from stress-relieving beverages to rejuvenating hair rinses. A bit of thanks for its popularity may be attributed to Beatrix Potter's charming story of Peter Rabbit, in which his mother serves a calming cup of chamomile tea after his frightening escape from Mr. McGregor. What child isn't eager to sip a cup, sweetened with honey, after hearing this story? And what mother isn't appreciative of the calming effect on her child!

With a variety of chamomiles, it can be difficult to choose which type to put in your herb garden. My choice is German chamomile *(M. recutita).* It is easier to grow from seed, has a more sturdy vertical growth habit, and is considered the best choice for medicinal value. With delicate, blue-green foliage and starry, white flowers blooming from June through frost, this 18- to 24-inch-tall feathery herb is a pretty sight.

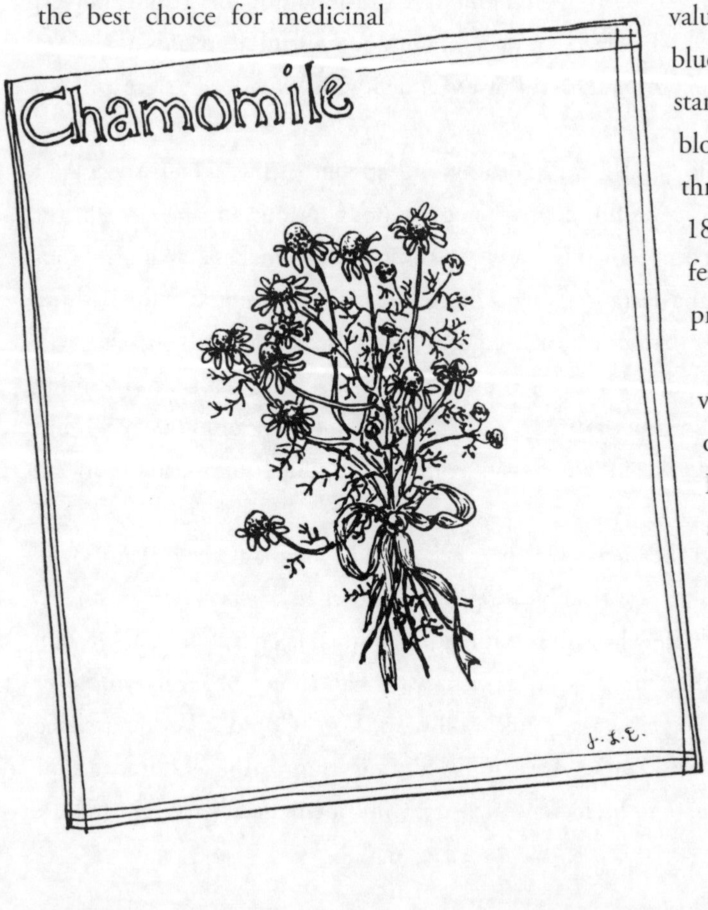

Chamomile is virtually carefree—once it's established! If your soil is heavy, simply work in some sandy loam. In late fall or early spring choose a mostly sunny spot for your chamomile bed, rough up the soil, and direct-sow seeds. If you sow in the fall, be sure to water your chamomile bed frequently in the spring until the seeds sprout. If sown in the spring, ditto: keep the seeds moist until they sprout. After seeds have germinated, provide light amounts of water.

The daisy-like flowers and flowering tops (two to three inches of the stems) are the part used. The flavor and scent of the flowers is somewhat like apples. Harvest throughout the blooming season. These may be used fresh or dried. It's best to dry them on a screen in a dark, dry, well-ventilated area, stirring frequently.

A few whole, fresh flowers and flowering stalks are pretty, flavorful, and healthful when tossed in a dinner salad. Dried flowers make a calming tea and are especially beneficial with a few mint leaves added and, after steeping, a bit of honey. This tea not only calms the nerves and helps relieve tension, it also treats stomachaches, heartburn, and indigestion, and is known to promote restful sleep.

Among its helpful properties, chamomile is anti-inflammatory; calms nerves, stress, and anxiety; eases headaches and pain; promotes restful sleep; aids digestion; and eases menstrual cramps. Dried flowers added with lavender in sleep pillows combine for a relaxing experience.

Chamomile is also useful for soothing and strengthening skin tissues. Add an infusion of chamomile flowers (strained) to body lotions and face cream for healthful results. Incorporate into soaps. A strong infusion makes a delightful foot soak to ease aches and fatigue. Warm, diluted tea is a soothing aid for bathing tired eyes. Added to shampoos, or used as a hair rinse, it's a tried-and-true way to reinvigorate limp, dull blond or brown hair. A soak in a bath after running hot water through a sachet of dried, crushed chamomile is not only relaxing, but can help to heal and calm inflamed skin. An infusion added to topical cream can reduce dermatitis.

Chamomile has other beneficial uses as well, and here's a story of my own. Working with children is a true blessing, but it poses risks, such as exposure to childhood illnesses! One who works with children must keep up on their vitamin supplements, as well as have home remedies on hand for whenever symptoms attack. Recently my eyes became pink, milky, and sore. Could it be the dreaded pinkeye (conjunctivitis) which was going around among the children at the weekly Bible school? I immediately turned to my medicinal herbs. Several are helpful in treating pinkeye and other eye ailments. From among them I chose chamomile. I made a strong tea with two tea bags and applied them to my sore eyelids as hot as I could stand (heat kills many of the microorganisms that cause pinkeye). Then I splashed my eyes with the warm tea. I also increased my vitamin C and zinc intake. I repeated the eye compress and wash several times a day. In about four days, whatever the problem was, it cleared up! A couple days later my eyes got rather milky again, so I repeated the procedure, with excellent results! I believe this simple treatment saved me the expense of a possible trip to the doctor, and cleared up the problem as quickly as with any prescription I've used!

Despite its myriad qualities, chamomile does have some cautions. This herb should be avoided by those who suffer from ragweed allergies—and, unfortunately, extended periods of daily consumption may lead to these allergies. Remember that chamomile is primarily a medicine, and medicines are used to treat problems—not to be daily consumed like water or food. Save that delicious tea for an evening when you are extra fatigued; toss those fresh flowers with your salad when you need a digestion booster; mix with skin cream when you feel the need to strengthen and refresh your skin. Proper use will endear this beneficial herb to you—misuse may do quite the opposite!

Tip

Chamomile is considered a beneficial neighbor to cabbage.

> *Lo, these are parts of [God's] ways: but how little a portion is heard of him? but the thunder of his power who can understand (Job 26:14)?*

CHICORY

(Cichorium intybus): Compositae family, perennial. Zones 3–10.

What a pretty sight! Exquisite blue flowers covering a tall, rangy plant in cheery profusion. Can that possibly be an herb? Yes, and a useful one too! Sometimes considered a weed, this hardy plant is a common sight along roadsides, in grassy areas, and where the ground has been disturbed. It has also found an important place in the garden—both medicinal and culinary—for centuries. Especially popular in Europe, its old English name is "succory."

Chicories comprise a genus that includes endive and escarole, peppery-tasting greens grown for steaming or adding to salads. Seed companies usually divide chicories into three groups: cutting chicories (the best loose-leaf variety), radicchio (which form small, tight heads resembling iceberg lettuce), and witloof chicory (traditionally grown for its roots). All have edible leaves that are sharp and bittersweet, but very healthful.

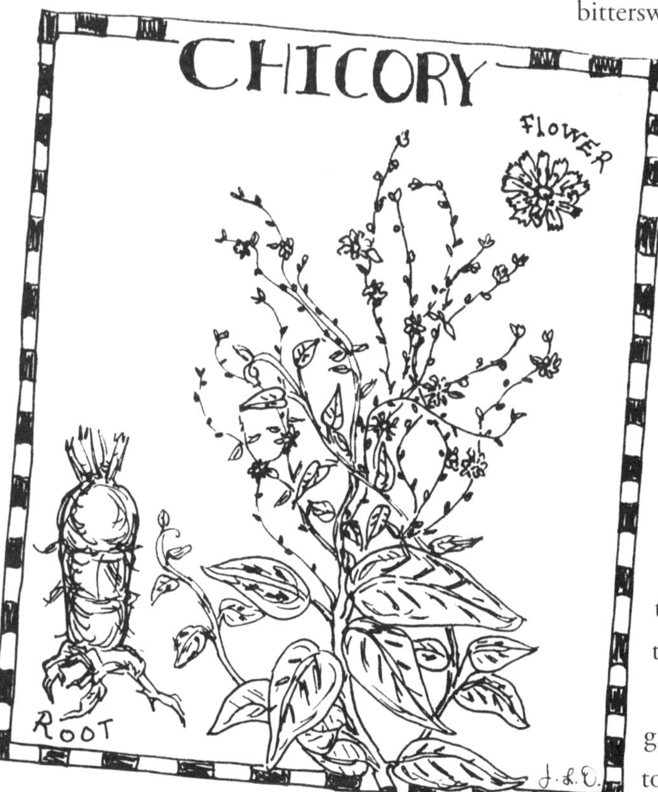

The first two tender perennials are typically grown as annuals, but witloof chicory is a hardy perennial in zones 3-10. We will be profiling witloof chicory (much like wild chicory) here. It is the most readily available of chicories grown especially for their roots—and to me, that's the best part!

Chicory is a tall-growing herb, having toothed lower leaves that resemble dandelions (except more bristly). Branched stalks with small upper leaves rise from the lower leaves, and in mid to late summer clusters of vibrant blue flowers burst into bloom. Chicory requires full sun, moderate water, and thrives in nearly any soil. In fact, it can easily take over, so keep an eye on it and be sure to thin regularly to keep in control. Sow seeds in early spring and, once the first true leaves appear, thin to about six inches apart. For the roots, cultivate much as you would carrots—but remember, witloof chicory tends to take over if left to itself! If you're after the leaves, treat rather more like spinach and harvest when young and tender.

The roots can be dug in early fall of the first year, or spring of the second. Leaves may be picked during the growing season, but are best early in the season while still tender. To dry leaves for tea, spread on screens and place in a dry, dark, well-ventilated area until they crumble easily. Store in an airtight container. You will be glad to know that the beautiful flowers of chicory are edible too. They make a lovely candied garnish, or a bright addition to salads. However, it is the young, peppery leaves and the mature roots that are most useful for medicinal purposes.

As mentioned previously, *C. intybus* has traditionally been grown for its roots. Dried, they can be ground into a flour and added (about one tablespoon per cup of all-purpose flour) to baked goods. The roots can also be dried, ground, and mixed with coffee to stretch it; or added to browned barley to make a delicious, healthful, 100% caffeine-free coffee substitute. Since picking the leaves hinders root development, I suggest growing a patch of witloof chicory for the roots, and another type (as an annual) for the young leaves.

It takes at least 100 days for the roots to be large enough to harvest, and they are even better after a year or two. After harvesting, wash well, slice thinly, and arrange (as with the leaves) on screens to dry thoroughly. Once the roots are dry, spread on a baking sheet and bake at 325 degrees for about half an hour. Don't let them scorch! Allow to cool, grind finely, and store in an airtight container. I suggest mixing with oven-browned ground barley for a satisfying hot beverage. Place a heaping teaspoonful in a cup, pour boiling water over it, mix well, and (if desired) add cream and sweetener. Delicious. And healthful too!

Witloof chicory is also known for blanched leaves. You may blanch, or "force," the roots to grow new leaf tops during the winter. These creamy white leaves are called "chicons," or "Belgian endive." Dig the roots in the fall, cut off the foliage, trim the bottom to about eight inches, and bury upright in a box of sand in a dark basement (or a warm greenhouse or shed, if you cover each buried root with an upside-down flower pot to keep out the light). Be sure to keep the area completely dark, since light will cause the leaves to turn green and become exceedingly bitter. Keep the temperature about 60 degrees. In three weeks new shoots—elongated and blanched—will have formed and be ready for the salad bowl or to be boiled or steamed. Serve with melted butter. A tasty treat—and you deserve it after all that effort!

Chicory leaves and roots both promote liver and gallbladder health. The tender young leaves (eaten or steeped in tea), or a drink made from the roots, make a good liver tonic. By improving bodily functions, yellow-hued eyes and skin may clear up. A drink made from the dried, roasted roots has been used to treat chronic constipation, give relief to those who have bilious attacks brought on by a sluggish liver or gallbladder, and is an overall tonic for digestive and urinary tract health. It is known to increase bile flow and reduce inflammation. Another interesting note is that the roasted roots are said to contain properties that kill bacteria. Oh yes, and if you are trying to eliminate coffee consumption, you might find this slightly bitter drink a good (and healthy!) substitute. You may also purchase ready-mixed drink powders containing chicory root at your health food store or Wal-Mart. Roma™ and Pero® are two excellent brands.

As a precautionary note, those who are anemic should consult a health care professional before using any part of the chicory plant. Also avoid it if you suffer from irritable bowel syndrome. Otherwise, chicory is a safe and healthy addition to your life.

Well, all of this sounds so good that I believe I'll go and make myself a steaming mug of dried, roasted chicory root! Care to join me?

Tips

Chicory greens and spent roots are considered good fodder for livestock.

Chicory is a good companion plant to plantain and clover in the herb garden.

COMFREY

(Symphytum officinale; S. x uplandicum): Boraginaceae family, perennial. Zones 3–9.

Comfrey is a plant both worthwhile and bothersome. Its looks are not against it, since the three- to four-foot-tall herb is showy and pretty. From April through September, it produces curved flower racemes (a bit like lily of the valley) of creamy to purple bell-like blossoms. The plant is thickly covered with broad, long, bright green leaves which are just a bit prickly to touch (and make your skin itch when you bruise them). The eight- to ten-inch-long lower leaves noticeably resemble a donkey's ears in shape and texture. The stems are hollow and bristly, and the roots thick, juicy, fleshy, and trailing. But don't let this rather lovely shrub deceive you; it can be terribly obnoxious if not contained!

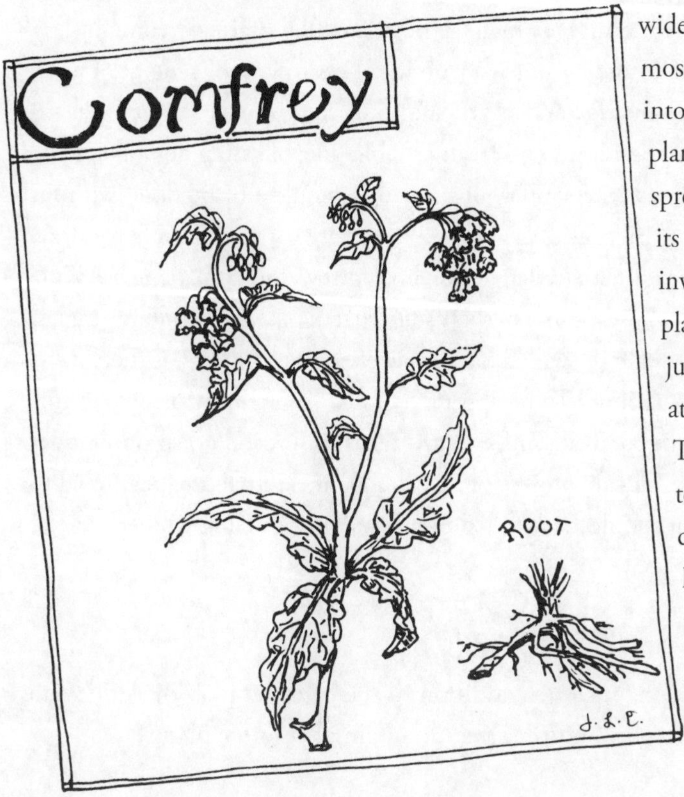

Comfrey prefers filtered sunshine; moist, rich, sweet soil; and thrives near streams, lakes, and ponds. Propagation from seed is difficult, so it is most often done (and easily!) through root division. This can be a bit *too* easy, since the simple act of using a tiller in your comfrey bed would cut up the roots and distribute them far and wide, where they would most certainly grow into new and vigorous plants. Each plant enjoys spreading itself out from its long root system, invading surrounding plants and making itself just a little too much at home anywhere! The best solution is to plant comfrey in deep sunken barrels or large pots equipped with drainage holes. And, even with its drawbacks, it is absolutely worth the extra effort to have this beneficial herb in your medicinal garden!

Harvest comfrey leaves just before the flowers bloom. Dig up the roots in the spring or fall with a garden fork. Both can be used fresh or dry (although the leaves lose some of their medicinal strength when dry) in poultices, compresses, infusions, decoctions, salves, and foot soaks. I suggest looking up a modern guide for using comfrey (written after the year 2010 by a professional herbalist) before extensive use of this powerful herb.

Traditionally, comfrey has been called "knitbone" or "bone set"—and with good reason. Of course it can't actually set bones or knit them back together, but both the roots and leaves contain a healing cell proliferant substance called allantoin. Allantoin is especially noted for soothing imflammation and reducing swelling around broken bones, increasing the speed of healing. A poultice of comfrey roots and/or leaves (using thin cotton to protect the skin from those irritating hairs on the leaves) also speeds healing of sprains, wounds, skin conditions, bedsores, bruises, bites and stings, inflamed bunions, burns, hemorrhoids, varicose veins, and leg ulcers. It eases joint pain and aching muscles too.

Incorporating infused comfrey (which has been carefully strained, removing any irritating hairs) into salves and creams is a wonderful treatment for acne, sunburns, excessively dry skin, dermatitis, and nearly any skin condition. I have also heard that it effectively stops nosebleeds and treats troubles like bleeding hemorrhoids.

Comfrey is sometimes taken internally, but this should not be done without careful research. As a precautionary note, there are two types of comfrey: *Symphytum x uplandicum,* also called Russian comfrey, and *S. officinale.* While both are safe for external uses, some herbals state that *S. officinale* contains higher levels of pyrrolizidine alkaloids, which have toxic effects on the liver. Others insist that it is the other way around! To be absolutely safe, I prefer only using comfrey externally. If you choose to take comfrey for internal purposes, do so only under the supervision of a health care professional. Infrequent external use is assumed to be perfectly safe, but it should be avoided by pregnant or nursing women.

Tip

The foliage of comfrey makes a rich addition to the compost pile. But don't add the root parts—unless you want to start a mountain of comfrey plants!

ECHINACEA

(Echinacea purpurea): Compositae family, perennial. Zones 3–9.

"Excuse me, but why do you have purple coneflowers in your medicinal herb garden? I thought they were wildflowers!" I'm glad you asked! This lovely prairie wildflower has its botanical name commonly found on labels of throat lozenges, immune system boosters, and natural respiratory products: echinacea.

Beneficial, as well as beautiful from head to toe, the whole of echinacea plants (fresh or dried) are used for tinctures, compresses, poultices, syrups, lozenges, infused honey and oil, ointments, salves, balms, and so much more! Of course, such a beauty isn't without value in your flower garden too! But I believe even a brief study of this powerful medicinal herb will encourage you to clear a space for it in your herb garden.

I prefer raising this hardy perennial from seed. Make sure the soil is well-drained and not too rich. In our cold climate, I simply rough up the soil in the fall, scatter seed, sift a thin layer of soil on top, and gently press down. Then all I have to do is wait until late spring when new echinacea plants are sure to greet me! In warmer climates, this won't be the best way. Sow seeds in early spring as soon as the ground can be worked. It helps if seeds are stratified for about a month in the refrigerator.

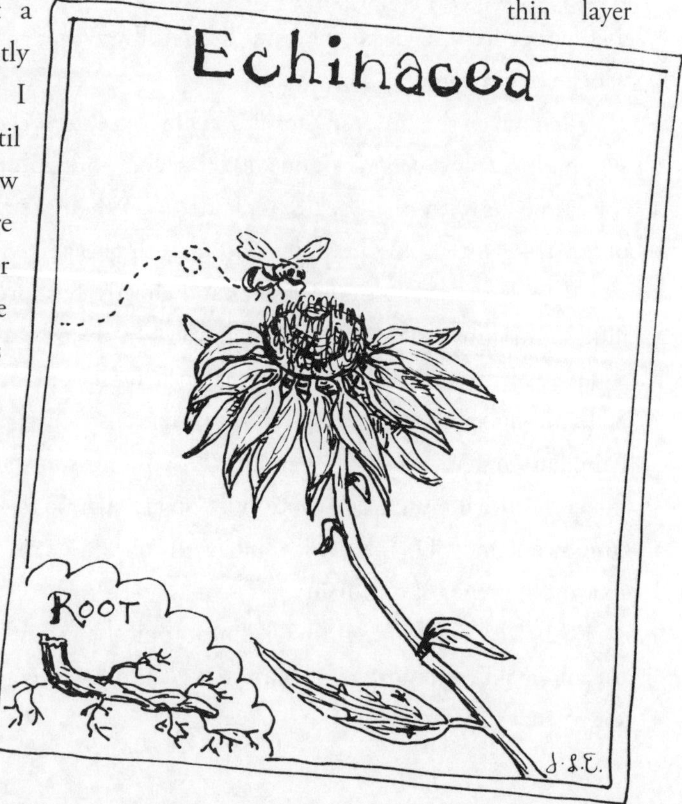

Since echinacea grows in clumps,

you can also divide the crowns of plants at least two years old (in cold climates, divide in the fall; in warmer climates, spring is best). Another option is to stop by a greenhouse in late spring and purchase echinacea seedlings. Be sure to purchase only those that are being sold as "herbs," not "flowers"—the flowers may have been treated with harmful chemicals not for consumption.

In mid to late summer, prepare yourself for a delightful glow of large purple to dark pink blossoms, lending an old-fashioned charm to your garden. Bees and butterflies love them! The flowers are unique, having many three-inch-long petals grouped around a cone-shaped center of dark reddish-orange. The stalks are sturdy and about two and one-half to three feet tall, with sparse, narrow, and hairy dark green leaves. Before the first frost hits, cut plants back to about two inches. After the first hard frost, mulch well. In the spring rake back the mulch and begin a moderate watering schedule.

Leaf parts, flowers, and seeds are harvested from the second growing season on. The roots are harvested in the fall or spring from mature plants of at least three years old. Whole plants are harvested when the flower is at its peak. All may be used either fresh or dried. Be sure to carefully research which parts are used for which applications.

When taken as a tea or in capsules, echinacea effectively stimulates the immune system. But only if you take it on and off, giving your body a break (say a two-week "off" time between one week of daily doses). When the first symptoms of a cold or flu strike, lozenges containing zinc and echinacea may be taken several times a day, stimulating the immune system and effectively shortening the length of the illness. This is my favorite use for echinacea—it always works wonders for me! But the uses of this excellent herb are many: it fights inflammation, fights bacterial and viral infection, treats respiratory troubles, is nourishing to the immune and lymphatic system, plus (as I mentioned) useful for shortening the length of colds, flu, and other illnesses. Use caution if you are allergic to ragweed or plants in the sunflower family. Do not use if you have autoimmune disorders. Some herbals say to avoid if pregnant or nursing.

Echinacea also shines in the realm of topical application. It promotes healing for minor skin wounds, acne, burns, sores, and has been found especially helpful for eczema sufferers.

Echinacea is in bloom close to the time calendula makes its sunny appearance. Combined, they make excellent topical applications, joining their healing properties. But that isn't all! I like to pick a bouquet of both flowers, adding their radiant beauty to a simple quart jar in the center of the kitchen table. What a cheery sight!

As a precautionary note: echinacea is helpful when used internally for a week or so, fighting a cold or boosting the immune system. But, as with all medicines, don't consume on a regular, uninterrupted basis. Your body will develop a tolerance for the herb, thus negating its medicinal effects.

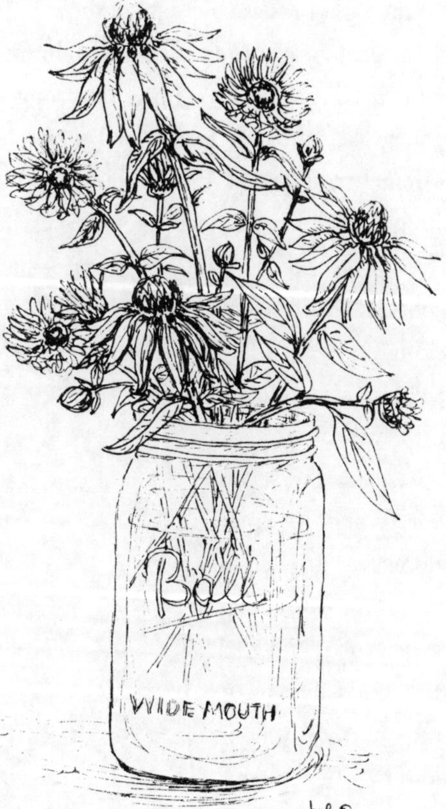

Tip

This tall, stately plant is best grown in wild herb fields, or positioned at the back of your herb garden so it won't shade other plants.

FLANNEL MULLEIN

(Verbascum thapsus): Scrophulariaceae family, biennial. Zones 3–9.

A familiar sight here in the southwest Rockies is that of small "forests" of four- to six and one-half-foot-tall mulleins. Growing in grassy fields, cropping up alongside roads, thriving among rocks, weeds, and disturbed areas, and voluntarily decorating the banks of streams and rivers, mulleins prove their hardy constitution by preferring rugged living conditions. They refuse to grow in tropical regions, but thrive in dry climates and poor soil.

The sight of these biennial herbs is impressive. Children especially are intrigued by the great height and amazing toughness of the plants. Knock one over, and it will immediately spring back into a standing position, apparently unharmed! The first year, mulleins merely form small rosettes of leaves. In the second year, a straight, extremely sturdy stalk rises high and is adorned with large (getting smaller as they climb the stalk), oval, silvery-green leaves that feel like soft flannel and are very durable. Tear a leaf, and the mild scent is reminiscent of spring greenery. The flavor is also mild and just a little bitter.

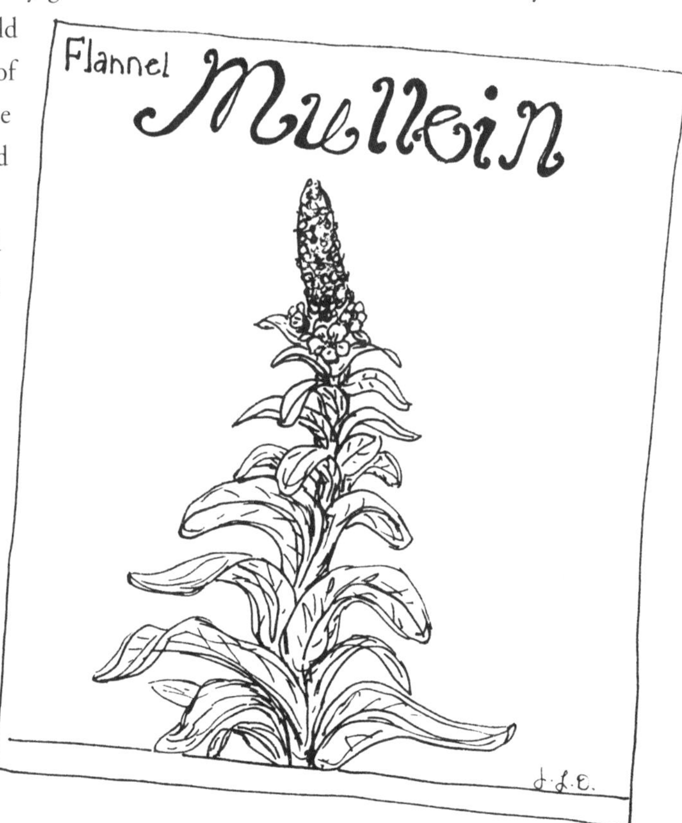

During the second year, when the plant shoots up in height, it produces a tall flower spike crowded with buds that open into buttery yellow flowers. These begin blooming at the bottom of the spike, and continue up to the tip over a period of a week or two.

Mulleins self-sow freely, but not always where you want them! I suggest taking pruning shears to the flower spike after you have harvested the delicate blossoms, preventing the plants from broadcasting their seeds. To save seeds for sowing where *you* want them, wait until the bright yellow flowers die and the spike begins to dry. Use pruning shears to snip off the spike. Place the spike upside-down in a large resealable plastic bag. Zip the top closed and shake gently. You'll be surprised at the hundreds of tiny black seeds (resembling snapdragon seeds) that are released! Save them to plant where desired in the fall or early spring.

In the medicinal herb garden, mullein makes a useful and attractive addition. Plant it among other herbs that prefer moderate water, full sun, and well-drained soil that isn't too rich. Place at the back of the garden where the giant herb won't shade other plants.

The roots, leaves, and flowers of mullein are all useful, fresh or dried, for medicinal purposes. Leaves may be harvested throughout the growing season. Roots are best harvested in the fall of the first year, or spring of the second. The flowers can be picked just as they bloom. All may be dried to preserve for winter, but use extra care drying the delicate flowers.

The roots of mullein are considered helpful for the urinary tract, working as a diuretic to relieve inflammation. The leaves and flowers are excellent for the respiratory tract and the skin. Mullein is soothing, as well as an emollient and astringent, and contains mild sedative properties.

Infused leaves or flowers help relieve coughs, chest colds, bronchitis, asthma, and diarrhea. Interestingly enough, infusions are also used to treat constipation. Be sure to strain out the hairy leaf particles when making infusions, syrups, balms, etc. These can be irritating and may cause rashes in some individuals. A tea is easier to take if infused in milk rather than water. Infused honey, or tea with honey added, can be used to remedy coughs. One effective topical application is to boil the leaves and use as a poultice for skin irritations (protect the skin from leaf hairs with a thin cotton cloth).

The pretty yellow flowers, picked just as they bloom and infused in olive oil, make a well-known topical treatment for reducing the pain and inflammation of earache. This infused oil is also useful when incorporated into ointments, creams, and salves for treating bruises, sores, insect bites, boils, and hemorrhoids. It is also said to be useful in healing skin damaged by frostbite.

Easy to grow, impressive to look at, and beneficial in so many ways—why not grow mullein in your own medicinal herb garden? I think you'll be glad you did!

Tip

Mulleins are a natural indicator of polluted soil. If they grow twisted, curly, or stunted, don't harvest from them! They may be contaminated by pollutants in the soil. Also, never harvest mulleins—even perfectly straight and healthy ones—that grow beside roads or in areas you know to be contaminated by insecticides or herbicides.

God

All of this grandeur that we see
Is simply but a glimpse,
A tiny portion, brief and small,
Of the wonder of Him.

The thunder of His awesome power
We cannot understand;
Yet every good and perfect gift—
It comes from His own hand!
–J.L.D.

HOREHOUND

(Marrubium vulgare): Labiatae family, perennial. Zones 3–8.

As a child, my knowledge of horehound was limited to those old-fashioned, slightly bitter, yet wonderfully yummy sticks of hard candy sold at a local gift shop. I always had a hard time choosing between the horehound sticks and the butterscotch. Usually horehound won the day! Despite the fact that some people grimace at the taste, after all these years I still favor it. Imagine my joy to find that horehound (and we're discussing *M. vulgare,* or white horehound, here) isn't merely a nice candy treat: it's a highly beneficial herb in the mint family! For centuries it has been a carefree addition to the medicinal herb garden.

A tough, sprawling, bushy herb, horehound requires full sun, but it isn't picky otherwise. It grows best in dry, sandy, rocky soil, and yet won't put up a fuss when placed in average garden soil (with a bit of gardening sand added) if allowed to dry between watering. Hot, full sun won't wilt horehound, so plant it where other herbs might shrivel or suffer heat stroke!

Propagate from seed by starting indoors and transplanting to the garden in mid to late spring. Root divisions work too, and sometimes tip cuttings, but that's a little more tricky. The leaves of this herb are small, oval, wrinkled with many veins, and are soft and

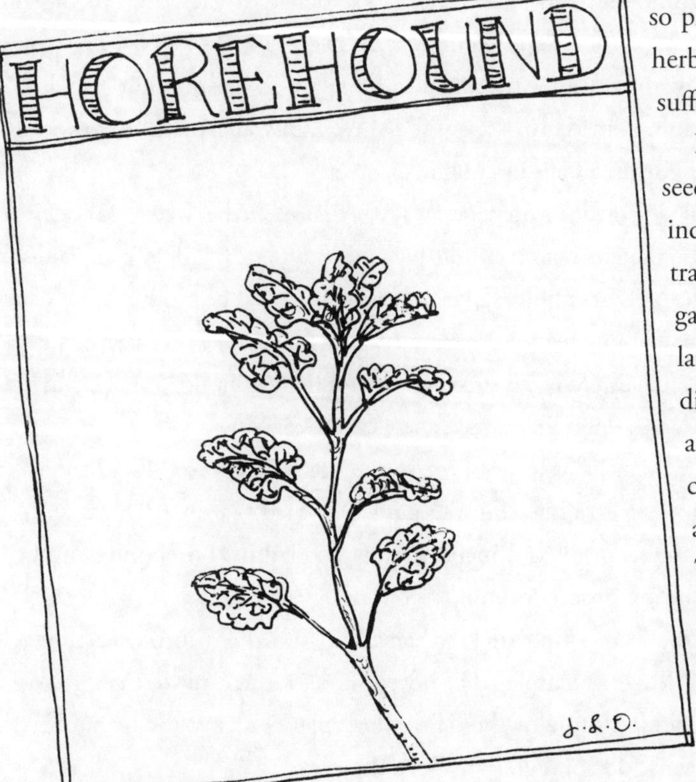

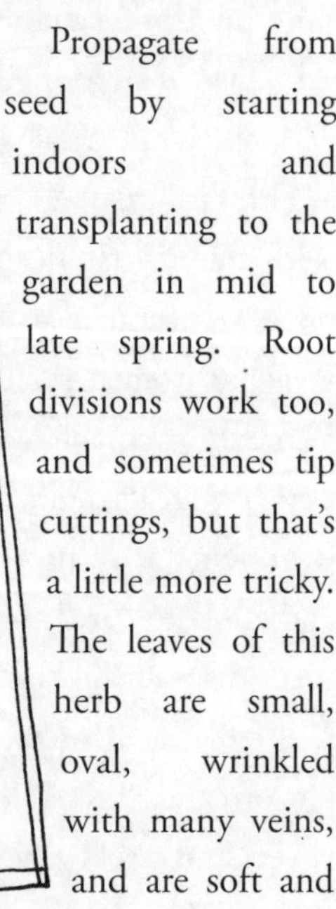

fuzzy to touch. They have a gray-green color with a frosty white velvet, especially on the underside of the leaves and along the woody stems and stalks, giving the plant its "white," frosted appearance. The scent is sharply sweet and the flavor, as we mentioned, bitter and uniquely its own. In the summer of the second year, watch for small, white, bee-attracting flowers that bloom in thick clusters along the stem. The leaves of this herb can be harvested at any time during the growing season. They may be used fresh or dried.

Horehound has been used for centuries to effectively treat coughs, bronchial and lung troubles, hay fever, sinusitis, and other respiratory problems. The leaves are effectively expectorant, helping clear the respiratory tract of mucus by promoting its ejection. Horehound also boosts the immune system and helps the body fight winter illnesses, plus it eases indigestion and bloating.

Horehound's presence in candy may be traced to early ways of preserving the bitter herb (cooked in sugar and made into disks) for use in treating the above-mentioned ailments. And that still works today! In fact, I've included several simple recipes in the recipe section. (See pages 153, 154 & 196.) You may also make syrups or infuse into honey to be taken in teaspoon doses while suffering from a cough. A medicinal-strength infusion in water makes a powerful gargle when suffering from a cold or cough.

Horehound can also be made into a potent tea (which needs to be sweetened), acting as a strong diuretic and therefore has traditionally been used to treat kidney complaints. Keep in mind that the herb has mild laxative properties too. And be cautious! In olden times, women used horehound tea to increase menstrual flow and expel the afterbirth. Pregnant women should carefully research (and consult their health care provider) before using horehound in doses that exceed a few candies or lozenges.

I have read that a weak infusion of horehound tea may be useful as a topical treatment for minor skin troubles. Simply pat the cooled tea on problem spots and allow to dry. Infused in oil and incorporated into balms, horehound can be used to speed the healing process of minor wounds.

I still reach for the horehound sticks whenever I find them in old-fashioned gift or candy shops! But I've learned that horehound is much more than a tasty sweet, and yes, I've added some of the hardy little plants to my medicinal herb garden! Why don't you add some to yours as well?

Tips

Some say that a container of strong horehound tea, placed in the middle of a picnic table, repels flies.

Horehound grows well when planted near thyme or rosemary. The result is pretty too!

HORSERADISH

(Armoracia rusticana): Cruciferae family, perennial. Zones 2–7.

If it wasn't for its medicinal properties, I doubt if horseradish would rate as an "herb of choice" in my estimation! Many disagree with me, but the powerfully hot, pungent taste of the roots and young leaves simply do not suit my palate. (Unless occasionally in the traditional Dresden sauce, or used sparingly in some types of mustards.) To add to that, I can't say that the rough, broad, bright green one- to three-foot elongated leaves are all that attractive either; and the clusters of tiny, four-petaled white flowers that top the plant in midsummer don't grab my attention.

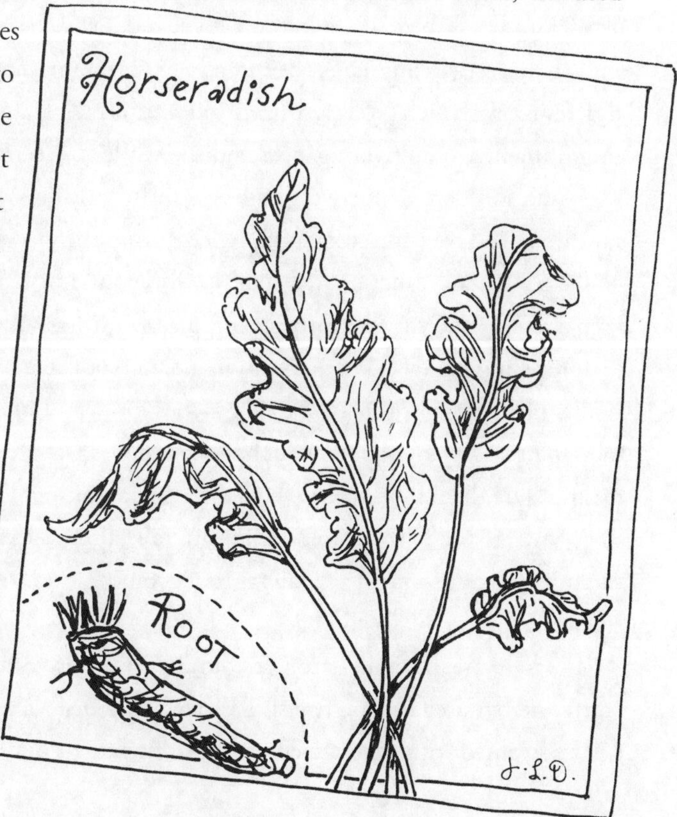

However, the fresh root treats a number of ailments, and is high in vitamins B and C; minerals calcium, phosphorus, sulfur, and iron; has antibiotic properties; and contains the amino acid asparagin, which is needed to maintain balance in the central nervous system. Well, after all of that, I just *couldn't* gallop past horseradish when deciding which herbs to include in this book! And if you enjoy the mighty flavor of this herb, be glad you do; it's good for you!!

Horseradish actually has nothing to do with horses. The name is thought either to come from the word "coarse," indicating its rough leaves; or from an English misinterpretation of the German word "meer" (meaning sea), to "mare," and then to "horse." It is in the same family as mustard and cress, and shares some of their medicinal qualities.

Horseradish is propagated by root cuttings. But beware! This herb spreads effortlessly and can overpower your garden in no time. The roots act much like comfrey roots, making themselves at home anywhere. If you accidentally broadcast roots in the soil by tilling, they will surprise you by sending up tough little plants where you least expect them! In fact, horseradish was called a "most pernicious weed" by a writer in the 1800s, and it *can* be ruinous if allowed to grow wild. I suggest sinking large, deep (at least 24-inch) containers into the ground and filling with rich, well-fertilized soil and a bit of sand. This creates an ideal environment for cultivating horseradish, while protecting other garden plants. Keep the soil damp (not wet) and be sure to position where there is plenty of sunshine. Add well-rotted manure twice during the growing season.

Once you have designated a place for your horseradish bed and carefully prepared the soil, in very early spring plant cuttings taken from a main taproot the preceding fall (and kept in sand in a dark, cool area over the winter). For best results plant straight roots about six inches long, and including the bud. Space a foot apart and plant about six inches deep (at a 45-degree angle, thicker end up), making sure the top is under two or three inches of soil. Pack soil firmly. Cut back the plants in the fall and mulch. In late fall (after several light frosts), you may carefully harvest some of the lateral roots coming from the main taproot. Return soil around main plant and pack firmly.

The roots are the main part used, but the young leaves are among the traditional "bitter herbs" used for the Jewish Passover. And believe me, they *are* bitter! These can be steamed with other greens to tone down their bite, but prepare yourself for a strong flavor. As a side note, be aware that the roots and leaves of horseradish are so biting-hot that they can produce sweating and cause heartburn. A Jewish doctor, an acquaintance of our family, says that at Passover celebrations older people are sometimes alarmed at the strong reactions to horseradish and think they are experiencing a heart attack. Not to worry! Horseradish is actually said to reduce high blood pressure.

As mentioned, you may harvest horseradish roots in the late fall of the first year, or midsummer from the second year on. The roots from one plant will typically be enough to make a half-pint of sauce, so you will need several plants if you want them for culinary as well as medicinal purposes. Horseradish is best stored in the refrigerator or buckets of dry, cool sand and used within three months. Remember that it will lose its flavor when exposed to sunlight, heat, or when cooked. For best results, use the roots fresh. For culinary purposes, grate fresh horseradish roots into sauces or mustards, lemon juices, vinegars, etc., and use within a day or two. You may also dry the roots, but it's much easier to purchase commercially prepared dried horseradish in the form of grains or flakes. Home drying seems to take the "punch" out of this herb.

As stated earlier, horseradish has important medicinal properties—especially when used to treat catarrhal (inflammation of the mucous membranes) and bronchial problems. In a glycerin tincture, it makes a tonic for bronchitis, plus lung and sinus congestion. This mixture is said to help fight whooping cough too. Another simple remedy for congestion is to grate the fresh roots and inhale the strong, almost overpowering aroma. This will clear congestion in a hurry! Grate a bit into green salads to boost the immune system. A rub made from avocado and grated horseradish is also excellent for treating chest colds.

Horseradish is good for digestive health as well. Eaten with rich, fatty foods, it aids digestion. Taken in a very weak tea, it works as a stimulant laxative (do not use on a regular basis). It is also extremely diuretic. Use sparingly—and I do mean sparingly—for these purposes!

Topically, horseradish has properties that relieve eczema and other skin troubles. Infuse grated roots in milk and splash over affected area for relief. Be sure to test on a small area first for sensitivity! This infusion stimulates circulation, so it is also beneficial for treating chilblains (painful, itchy inflammation usually affecting the toes, fingers, and external parts of the ears, and caused by exposure to cold), cold feet, and achy joints. A poultice of grated roots directly applied speeds the healing of boils.

Use caution when working with horseradish. Some find that grating it irritates their eyes to an exceedingly painful extent (worse than slicing onions). Also, only use sparingly and with caution for internal purposes; large doses can cause inflammation of the lining of the throat and stomach.

Despite its rough appearance, powerful scent and flavor, and overbearing growth habits, I think you'll agree that horseradish has enough redeeming qualities to find a place in the herb garden!

Tip

Horseradish is said to repel the Colorado potato beetle. Why not sink a few barrels around the parameter of your potato patch?

It will not be enough to tell people we are Christians—they will wait to see the evidence of it in our lives. –J.R. Miller

LAVENDER

(Lavandula angustifolia): Labiatae family, perennial. Zones 6–8.

Spicy-sweet with an aroma all its own, few fragrances are as pleasant as that of English lavender. No wonder it shows up in lotions, soaps, body washes, shampoos, bath sachets, and a myriad of other skin and body care products. Not to mention its delightful presence in potpourri mixes, candles, and room fresheners. But the fragrance, though therapeutic in calming nerves and tension, is merely a fragment of the wonder of this herb. Its healing and mild antiseptic properties for skin ailments, cuts and scrapes, sunburns, and insect bites make it a good choice for your medicinal herb garden.

English lavender is a beautiful, bushy shrub that reaches nearly three feet in height. The pointed leaves are silvery, pale green, and loaded with fragrance. Rub a leaf between your fingers to release the oils, and breathe deeply of the sweet, clean, fresh, and calming perfume. The flowers range from pale lavender to deep purple, covering the top two or three inches of the tall, spiky stems with a lovely mist of color in midsummer. Before the first frost in cold climates, or in the early spring where it's warmer, prune bushes to about three inches above the ground. In the spring, rake away dead leaves and watch for new growth!

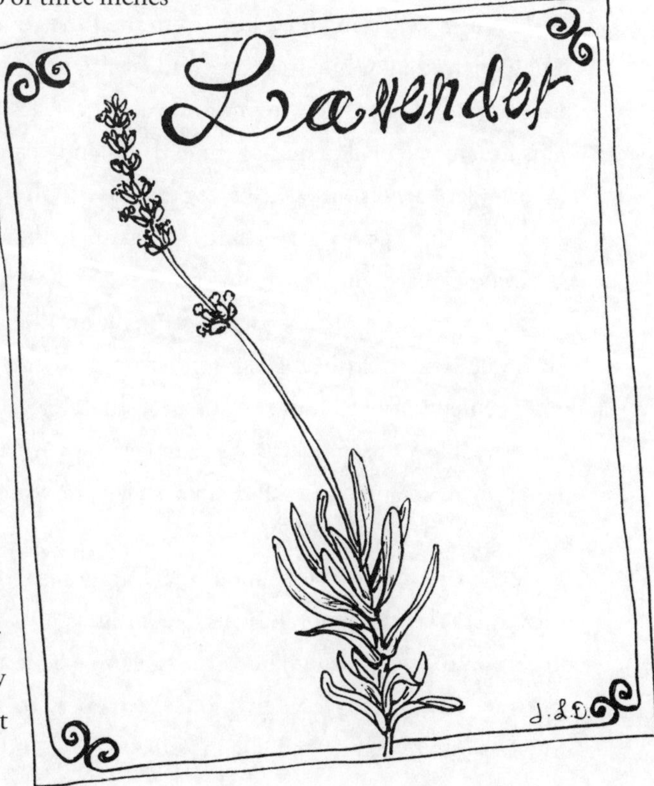

Because of its breathtaking beauty, wonderful fragrance, and low-maintenance, flower gardeners often grow lavender just for its looks. It simply requires well-drained sandy soil, a little water, and lots of sunshine to thrive. And it makes a nice container herb, too, if planted in a large pot equipped with drainage holes and a good potting mix. Add a bit of perlite and gardening sand for best results. Move the pot to catch the sun, water sparingly, and watch your lavender flourish! Lavender is most easily propagated by cuttings and root divisions. If you live in a harsh climate, cut your plants back and mulch well in the fall.

As a medicinal herb, the leaves and flowers alike are used for therapeutic, skin care, and home care purposes. Harvest early in the day directly after the flowers open, as that's when the oil content is highest, and before the sun has sapped the volatile essence. It's best to choose a dry morning for harvest, and then tie bunches of lavender and hang in a dark, dry, well-ventilated place to dry. Since the essential oil derived from lavender is extremely potent, professional herbalists caution that it should not be used during pregnancy or taken internally.

Who doesn't enjoy dried lavender sachets?! Well, the answer is, moths and other pests! Hang a sachet in your closet to freshen the air and repel wool moths. Place among linens for a subtle fragrance and, again, protection from moths. Add dried rosemary, mint, tansy, and thyme and tuck into chests where you plan on storing items for an extended period of time; this blend gives even more protection.

Lavender sachets are also known to soothe the nerves and promote restful sleep. Place one under the faucet for a relaxing bath before bed. Incorporate into a sleep pillow, where the heat from your head will release lavender's restful essence.

The essential oil of lavender is strongly antifungal and antibacterial. A dab on simple household burns, sunburns, or cuts and scrapes eliminates pain and helps tremendously to heal skin tissue. Mix a few drops of lavender essential oil into olive oil to rub into varicose veins, or to treat bruises. Dilute in aloe vera gel and apply to scraped knees and elbows! This mixture promotes healing of minor wounds.

And I have my own story about that! Not long ago, while getting a Bible lesson ready for a class of children, I needed to move a table so I could tape Scripture posters on the wall. As I grabbed the table to give it a pull—ouch! My fingers slid across a sharp metal piece, giving me some very painful slices. All I had time to do was wash my hands and wrap the cuts with Band-Aids®. But once I got home two hours later, I decided to see what lavender essential oil can do. I stirred about ten drops into a small basin of warm water and swished my throbbing fingers in it for about thirty seconds. It did relieve the pain! Then I let the cuts dry completely and later applied a mixture of a dab of thick aloe vera gel (the type that's labeled "After-Sun Gel") and a strong dose of lavender oil on the cuts, wrapping them with more Band-Aids®. I repeated this for three nights, letting the cuts dry off and on during the day. By then, the cuts were almost completely healed! In a week, all I could see were faint lines where the cuts had been. And there was very little dead skin to clip off! I certainly was pleased with the results! Now I keep a one-ounce bottle of oil diluted in aloe vera, ready for emergencies!

If you suffer from rashes, acne, or other skin irritations, why settle for drugs that pose health risks? Dilute lavender essential oil in aloe vera gel or a gentle cream. Test on the inside of your elbow first, and if no irritation occurs, apply liberally on the affected area daily. Reducing inflammation, healing skin tissue, cleansing the skin, and adding a subtle, calming fragrance all at once—what a delightful remedy!

A dab of undiluted essential oil on insect bites relieves the itch and calms the pain. Lavender is also excellent for treating tension headaches. Rest your head on a small pillow filled with dried lavender (and, if desired, sprinkle the lavender with essential oil before closing the pillow), or make a fabric eye mask stuffed with the same. This can chase away a headache and calm nerves. Or simply use one of the pillows when you take your next nap! It is delightfully relaxing.

As a precautionary note, in rare cases lavender (especially the essential oil) can cause allergic reactions such as (surprisingly!) headaches, rashes, and respiratory troubles. Be cautious and start off sparingly. If any adverse reactions occur, discontinue use.

For me, even the looks of lavender in bloom, such a soft, gentle sight, is calming to the nerves. Plant some in your garden and see if you agree!

Tips

Plant lavender in pots on your deck. You will love the fragrance, but mosquitoes don't!

When lavender blooms, bees are sure to follow!

LEMON BALM

(Melissa officinalis): Labiatae family, perennial. Zones 4–10.

Lemon balm is a favorite plant for the herb garden, and not necessarily due to its looks. Some consider the bushy low-growing herb (which resembles a small-leaved nettle) too weedy in appearance to make a pretty sight. Others insist that the mint-like, heart-shaped, dark green leaves are lovely—especially in June when clusters of tiny, creamy white flowers discreetly adorn the top of the flowering stalks. Regardless of differing opinions about the appearance of lemon balm, most folks agree that the luscious minty-lemon fragrance, heralding the same delightful flavor, makes lemon balm a must for the garden.

Lemon balm is one of those herbs that is super-easy to care for. It doesn't complain over poor soil, thrives in full or partial sun, won't spread by runners and overtake surrounding plants, and is cold tolerant (though it must be protected from frost). It also makes an excellent container herb if planted alone in a large, well-drained pot.

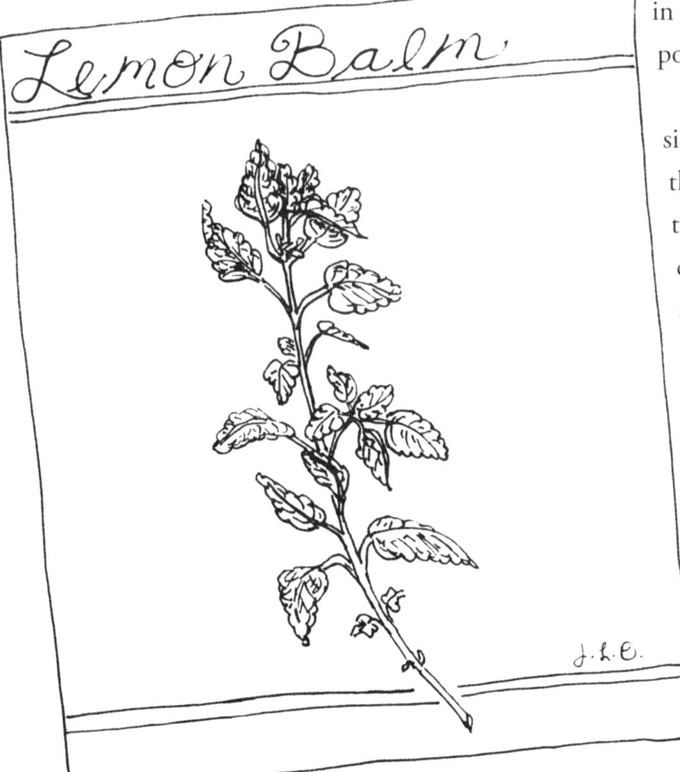

Propagation is simple: divide the thick root clumps in the spring or fall, take cuttings, or plant the seeds. One caution: lemon balm self-seeds freely. Remove spent flowers before the seeds fall.

You may trim lemon balm vigorously without harming it—which is something you'll find yourself doing often once you're accustomed to using the wonderful leaves! To encourage new, lush growth, cut the whole plant down to about five inches high just after the flowering stalks shoot up. (Don't discard the leaves—you'll find many uses for them!) However, be sure to allow a few stalks to flower. Bees (especially honeybees) revel in the nectar-laden blossoms, which makes a delicious honey. This accounts for the plant's generic name, *Melissa,* which comes from the Greek word "bee." In fact, early beekeepers planted lemon balm around their beehives, believing the delightful fragrance kept the honeybees from swarming. Some fruit growers plant lemon balm among their orchards to attract bees to pollinate the fruit trees.

Lemon balm is best used fresh from the plant. You may keep a few sprigs in a bit of water in the refrigerator for two or three days, but otherwise I don't recommend storing this herb. The only exception is to dry for use in sachets.

As so often happens with herbs, lemon balm can fit well into both the culinary and medicinal categories. It is especially popular as a flavorful and refreshing tea, served hot or iced and sometimes steeped with mint leaves. You can also use the tea (with a pretty leaf added) to make elegant ice cubes or ice rings for large bowls of citrus-flavored drinks.

With their bold lemon taste, the leaves are just wonderful added fresh to fruit salads, smoothies, desserts, and used as edible garnishes. You may substitute lemon balm in any recipe that calls for mint, use chopped leaves in place of lemon zest, add the cooled tea to lemonade as part of the liquid, and make a gentle flavoring for ice cream and frosting by using a few drops (or more!) of a strong infusion made of the leaves simmered in a small amount of water, then strained. Speaking of ice cream, go ahead and add a tablespoon of the fresh chopped leaves to your ingredient list along with the infused flavoring. It's so refreshing and lends a pretty pale green color.

Lemon balm is also tasty added to certain types of soup (mainly seafood), salad dressings, sauces (especially served over fish), green salads, and egg dishes. Want a taste-adventure? Add some leaves to carrots the next time you steam them, toss in melted butter, and serve alongside fish, seafood, or chicken dishes. Yummy!

But now you're looking up the section heading and wondering, *"Medicinal?* Why is lemon balm in *this* section, anyway? It sounds like it shines in culinary uses." I'll explain!

Lemon balm leaves are more than just flavorful and fragrant. They contain gentle healing essences which have medicinal properties for both external and internal ailments. Best known as a mild tranquilizer, it makes a good bedtime tea, or added (dried) to a lavender sleep pillow or bath sachet. It is also reputed to lower blood pressure, calm heart spasms, and treat colic and nervous stomach.

Lemon balm is wonderful infused in honey or syrups, making a delicious treatment for sore throats, coughs, and colds. Due to its gentle reputation, it is often recommended for children's health. This herb is beneficial for maintaining digestive health, strengthening the immune system, battling winter illnesses, treating pain (infused in olive oil, it makes an effective massage oil for aching muscles), and it helps strengthen the nervous system.

Lemon balm is an excellent stress, tension, and headache reliever. It is both relaxing and rejuvenating. The tea (especially when taken hot) induces sweating, helping lower high body temperatures caused by hot weather, overexertion, or a fever. Lemon balm has antioxidant properties, making it a healthful addition to your daily diet. It contains an antiviral agent as well, which fights mumps, cold sores, fever blisters, and other viruses. Chew a few leaves or use an infusion as a mouthwash to freshen your breath.

And who could ignore lemon balm's excellent topical uses? Infuse in water and use as a cleansing facial rinse. Its antihistamine action treats eczema, insect bites, and wounds. Incorporate infused oils into ointments. Use dried leaves in bath sachets for an overall skin cleanser and refresher. Use in compresses and poultices for slight wounds or skin disorders. And the list goes on!

Gentle and effective for overall health, now you see why I couldn't resist putting lemon balm under the "medicinal" category!

Precautionary Note: Lemon balm can slightly inhibit the thyroid-stimulating hormone. If you have thyroid problems, consult your health care provider concerning use of lemon balm. If you do not suffer from thyroid troubles, lemon balm is considered gentle and safe for frequent use.

LEMONGRASS

(Cymbopogon citratus) Gramineae family, perennial. Zones 8–11.

Some call its appearance unkempt, but I think the rough, narrow, slightly sticky leaves of lemongrass make a graceful shape, bending down at the ends and hanging charmingly over the rim of a large terra-cotta pot. At certain times of the year the leaves take on a pretty rust color at the tips, contrasting delightfully with the pale green of the rest of the leaf. But regardless of how much you like (or dislike!) the plant's appearance, tear off a leaf, take a deep breath, then put your tongue on the cut edge. Wonderful! The delicious fragrance and distinct flavor of lemon make the herb a general favorite.

Lemongrass grows in a bushy clump, getting larger every year in zones 8-11, sometimes reaching four feet in height. It prefers hot and moist climates, but rather sandy, well-drained soil. In colder zones, lemongrass acts as an annual and is much smaller. Here in southwest Colorado, it makes an especially nice potted plant—*if* kept well-watered, frequently misted, and placed in a sunny spot on the deck. Some keep a bush in their heated greenhouses, where it is said to grow almost as hardily as in its native climate of India and Sri Lanka.

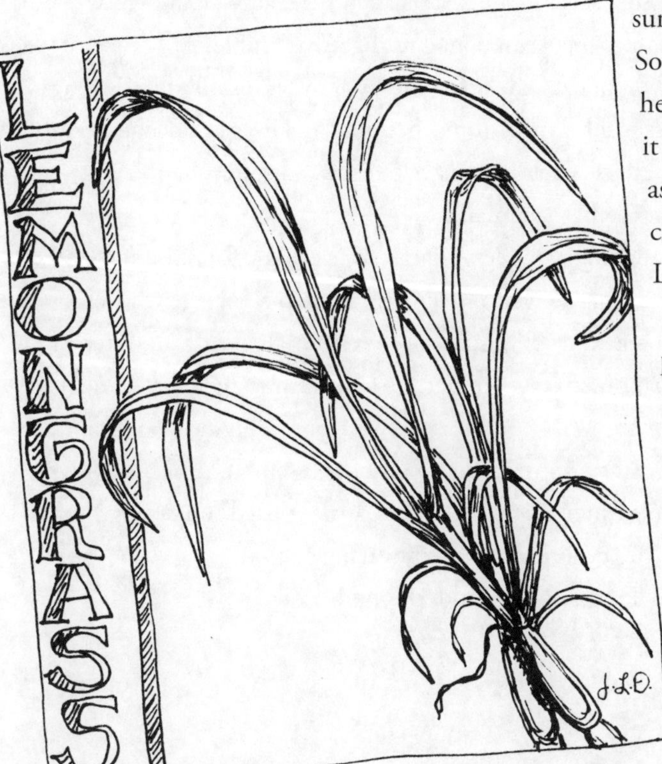

Lemongrass is best propagated by dividing the roots in the spring. Be careful to protect the main root system of the parent plant. Place new divisions directly into prepared ground, firm the soil, and keep very moist until established. Seeds work too, but require more effort. Start them in a greenhouse, or (in hot, moist climates) outdoors after all danger of frost. Once established, water regularly but don't allow soil to get soggy. Lemongrass benefits from frequent trimming to make room for new growth. In the fall, cut down to about three inches above the ground.

Popular in Asian cuisine, the distinct flavor of lemongrass is also used to flavor ice cream, candy, and pastries. The steeped leaves make a superbly refreshing tea (hot or cold!), and lend a delicious taste to steamed or simmered fish and chicken when added to the water (discard leaves before serving). Lemongrass is considered a medicinal food and is used by chefs who specialize in preparing such foods.

As a medicinal herb, lemongrass is amazing—see if you don't agree! It acts as an astringent, tonic, and aid for digestion. It contains many nutrients, including calcium, iron, magnesium, manganese, phosphorus, potassium, selenium, and zinc. The leaves can be used fresh or dried in teas, infusions, tablets, infused honey or oil, and also work well in sleep pillows and bath sachets.

Sipping tea made from the leaves isn't just a pleasant beverage—lemongrass tea is used to treat fevers, irregular menstruation, and digestive problems. It combats the flu and common cold, boosts the immune system, is useful for healing intestinal irritations and soothing the stomach lining, relieves headaches, and has a delightfully cooling effect when you get overheated (as often happens after spending a day working in the herb garden!).

Used both internally and topically, lemongrass is excellent for skin and nail health. Taking a course of tea or tablets has been said to help teenagers who suffer from oily skin and acne. If you add a few drops of the essential oil to bath water, or tie a sachet of the dried, crumbled leaves under the faucet, the beneficial elements are readily absorbed when the warm bath opens your pores, giving you a faint, fresh lemon scent and acting as a natural deodorant. The essential oil also destroys many forms of bacteria and fungi, and is a good treatment used full-strength on ringworm, or to promote the healing of bruised or damaged skin.

Don't you agree that lemongrass is a wonderful herb?!

Tip

Lemongrass is said to be a fly, flea, and mosquito repellent, making it a useful as well as decorative addition to your deck or patio. Infused in olive oil and dabbed on the skin, it keeps those pests directly away from you as well! Be sure to keep the infused oil away from eyes, mucous membranes, and sensitive areas.

PEPPERMINT

(Mentha x piperita): Labiatae family, perennial. Zones 5–9.

Just how many uses does peppermint have? Stop for a minute and think of all the products you have on hand right now that contain this versatile herb! It can be found in candies, chewing gum, breath fresheners, toothpaste and dental products, after-dinner mints, herbal teas, hand and body soap, bubble bath, cough drops, lip balm, balm for sore muscles, antiseptic creams, room fresheners, household cleaning products, and more! Whether we realize it or not, the flowering tops, oil, or leaves are an important ingredient in many products we use every day.

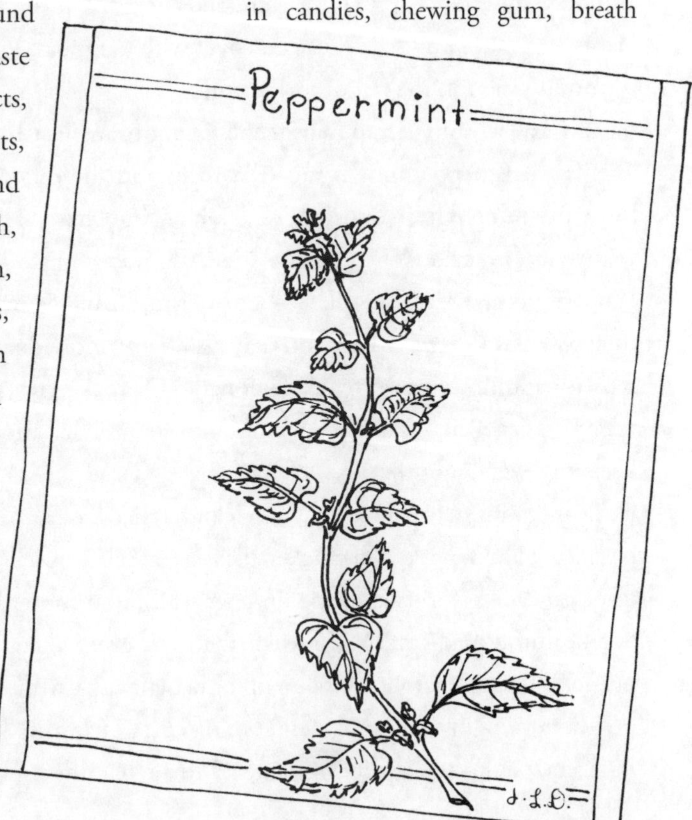

Peppermint is a hybrid cross between *M. aquatica* (water mint) and *M. spicata* (spearmint). It is a hardy, beautiful plant with a spreading habit that makes planting in pots or sunken containers desirable—unless you want peppermint as a deliciously fragrant ground cover! This vigorous herb thrives in full or partial sun; likes slightly acid, moderately rich, moist soil (but will grow in just about any soil!); and benefits from having its leaves picked frequently. And that's easy to do, since there are so many uses for them!

Reaching about three feet in height, the dark stems are covered with purple-edged, dark green, lance-shaped leaves that are smooth, but serrated around the edges. They contain the aromatic oil menthol, which is the basis for this herb's healing potential. The fragrance is strong like all mints, but peculiar to itself. Pick a leaf, rub it between your fingers, and immediately you'll say, "Peppermint!" This is, of course, the herb from which peppermint oil is obtained.

In midsummer, spikes of small, lilac-pink flowers begin blooming. To prevent a spindly appearance, pinch the stem ends in early spring. In the fall, prune back plants to about two inches tall and cover with compost. Propagation is best done by root division in the fall or early spring.

To harvest, cut the top half of the young stems just before the plant flowers. This is when peppermint is most flavorful and the oil content at its peak. The leaves can be used fresh or dried. To dry, hang bunches of leafy stems in a dark, dry, well-ventilated area. When crisply dried, crumble and store in airtight containers. Peppermint also freezes well. A good way to do this is by first wrapping in foil, then sealing in a freezer bag. You may also freeze individual leaves in ice cubes for a pretty addition to iced tea or lemonade. Or make crystallized mint leaves (see recipe on page 154—same procedure as crystallized horehound leaves), which will keep for several months.

Peppermint may find its way into candies; ice cream; desserts; jams and jellies; beverages; lamb, pork, and chicken dishes; leaf salads; used as garnishes; made into tasty pancake syrup (see recipe on page 188); and more. But it works primarily as a healthful medicinal herb. Medicinal, yes, even when we're using it for other purposes! See if the following lineup of benefits isn't wonderful:

The revivifying flavor of peppermint comes from its high menthol content. A steam made by simmering water with a handful of peppermint leaves, or two drops of peppermint oil, is excellent for relieving congestion and tension headaches. Leaves brewed into a tasty tea and served hot or iced will gently relieve indigestion, relax the muscles of the digestive tract, ease menstrual cramps, and quiet nerves. It stimulates bile secretion, and can be used to treat irritable bowel syndrome.

Menthol kills bacteria, parasites, or viruses that may be in the stomach and intestines. It battles fungus infections, relieves heavy colds due to its decongestant action, can be used as an effective chest rub to relieve respiratory problems, and builds the immune system! In fact, it is said that drinking at least one cup of peppermint tea a day through the winter will help keep away the common cold.

Peppermint is also a good treatment for chills, colic, diarrhea, headache, and nausea. Balms and liniments made with peppermint essential oil are excellent for easing rheumatism and muscle spasms. A hot bath with either a bath sachet of dried peppermint leaves (or a few crushed fresh leaves) or several drops of peppermint oil is cleansing, soothing, and an effective tension-tamer.

Peppermint is loaded with nutrients, vitamins, and minerals as well, which combine to promote overall health. Truly it is an amazing herb!

Of course, an herb as potent as peppermint has its cautions. It is said that pure peppermint oil may interfere with iron absorption, and should be avoided by nursing mothers, people with gallstones, and those who suffer from gastroesophageal reflux or similar conditions. Also, pure peppermint essential oil can be lethal—do not ingest more than a very tiny amount! Remember, when used as a flavoring a drop or two flavors a *whole batch*—not just one serving! If you happen to get peppermint oil in your eyes or a cut, wash immediately with whole milk; the fat binds with the oils, relieving pain.

Peppermint extract is perhaps a safer choice for cooking purposes than the essential oil. The difference between pure essential oils and extracts is simply this: pure essential oil is distilled from the plant and therefore highly concentrated; extracts are a mixture of the essential oils suspended in alcohol or some other base, which dilutes them for use in flavoring candies and foods.

Blending peppermint leaves with other herbs, such as oregano, echinacea, and mullein, makes a healing drink for respiratory troubles. In fact, peppermint leaves are a nice base for many herbal teas to treat varied ailments. I especially like to blend the leaves with chamomile, lemon thyme, lime basil, and red raspberry. Yum!

And that about wraps up the profile of this excellent herb. Now I think I'll go brew a cup of tea—peppermint, of course!

Tips

Peppermint oil is so strong, it sends mice running! Mix a few drops in water and keep an open container under counters or in attics. Even a few sprigs of dried peppermint seem to do the trick!

The mint family repels aphids, cabbage moths, and Colorado potato beetles.

Stinging nettle grown nearby is said to promote the production of oil in peppermint. Chamomile, however, has the opposite effect!

PLANTAIN

(Plantago major; P. lanceolata; P. media): Plantaginaceae family, perennial. Zones 3–9.

Growing up in a mountainous area in southern California, wild plantain flourished like a weed in the dry clay soil of our yard. It also abounded along hiking trails and stream banks. Reaching about 10 to 24 inches tall, I always liked the unique look of it—so different from other weeds. At one time, we didn't realize what the plant was. My older brother and I enjoyed picking the tall, skinny, leather-like green stalks, popping the fuzzy white and tan flowerheads off, and weaving the stalks into little mats and baskets.

The long, narrow, glossy leaves of that variety *(P. lanceolata)* were tough and had predominant ridges that gave them a distinctive look among the surrounding weeds. To me, the flowerheads in delicate bloom resembled little bees with their wings fluttering. Too bad I didn't know then (when unsuspecting barefoot toes sometimes stepped on unsuspecting bees hovering among the clover) what wonderful uses plantain leaves have for treating bee stings!

As with many herbs, plantain comes in a variety of types—making it hard to choose which one to put in your herb garden! I decided to focus on the three most widely known varieties.

So far as looks go, I still like *P. lanceolata* the best (probably because it reminds me of my childhood). *P. major* is quite different in appearance, having broad, heavily veined leaves (that are tasty and nutritious picked young and tossed in salads!) and long greenish spikes of flowers that bloom in midsummer. It is shorter (about eight to twelve inches tall) and a more unkempt sight. Lastly, the *P. media* is especially well known for its leaves' styptic effect (helping to stop bleeding) on minor wounds.

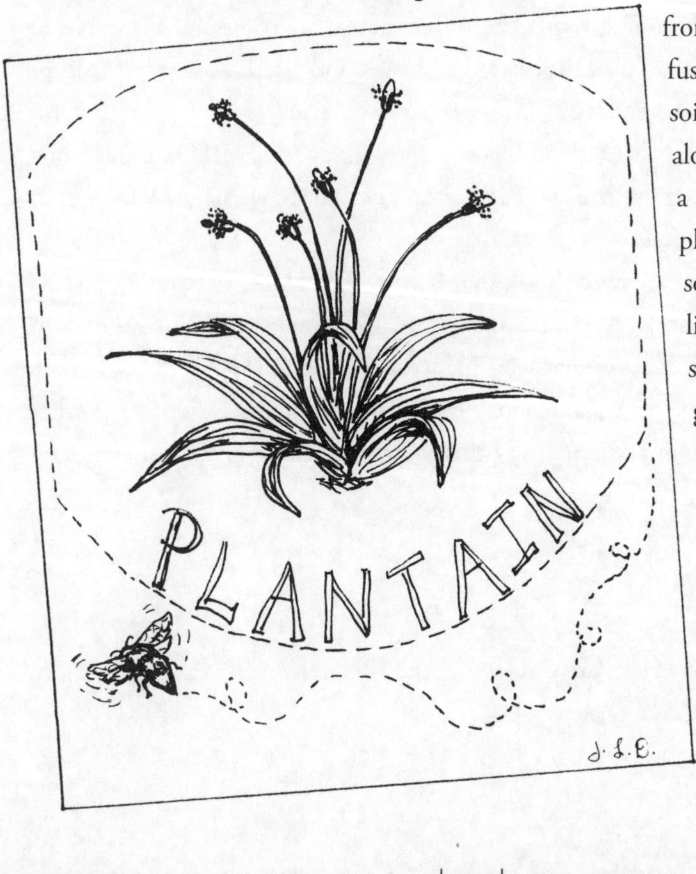

Plantain grows in clumps and should be spaced about a foot apart, although it doesn't seem to mind crowding. All three varieties grow easily from seed and aren't fussy. They brave clay soil, and yet thrive along the banks of a stream. However, plantain does have some preferences! It likes full or filtered sun and won't germinate unless the soil temperature is about 60 degrees. Water moderately after seeds sprout. Surprisingly, if you decide to plant this herb in a pot with rich soil, it will astound you with its lush, bushy appearance!

The whole of plantain can be harvested just after the flowers die and the seeds are easily brushed from the flowerheads. Discard the leathery stalks and use fresh, or dry the rest of the plant (including the roots). Research each part's use, and use (or store and label) accordingly.

Each variety of plantain has benefits in common: the leaves contain healing, antibiotic, and antiseptic properties that are truly wonderful when applied to blisters, bee or insect stings or bites, slight wounds, and sores. If you are working in the yard, on a picnic, or taking a hike and don't have your first-aid kit handy, plantain grows wild in most grassy places in zones 3–9. Simply search out a plant, apply the bruised leaves (bruise by chewing lightly) to insect bites, stings, burns, minor wounds, or blisters—and find quick relief! Immediate application speeds up the healing process. In fact, I've read that when suffering from a blister on a long hike, you can quickly mash a leaf and apply it to the blister, affixing with first-aid tape. Then continue your hike with minimal discomfort!

Bites, stings, and wounds aren't the only troubles that respond favorably to plantain. You can make an infusion of the leaves and use it topically to deep-cleanse the skin, or take a weak infusion as an internal tonic (sparingly!) for indigestion, heartburn, thrush, and bladder and kidney troubles. On a side note, probably all of us recognize the seeds of *P. ovata* (psyllium), which are widely used as a bulk-forming laxative.

I suggest finding a reference book that thoroughly addresses plantain and its uses before experimenting. Also, find quality pictures to help you identify different varieties of this herb. Be sure that wild plant in your back yard *really* is plantain before using it! Some types resemble foxglove (which has major cautions!) or other dangerous plants. Enjoy the benefits of this soothing, healing herb, but be careful and be wise!

Tip

Plant beside hyssop; the uses are similar and they like each other's company! Both herbs also do well in rock gardens.

ROSEMARY

(Rosmarinus officinalis): Labiatae family, tender perennial. Zones 8–11.

Picture for a minute the beautiful sandy shores of the Mediterranean Sea. Full sun beats down on hot sand. The air is full of an invigorating humidity misting from the sea. Take a deeper breath. Yes, there's a hint of pine scent on the salty breeze, mingled with a minty, sage-like aroma. It's coming from those bushy, gray-green six-foot-tall shrubs covered with leaves that resemble spruce needles and gorgeous little lavender-blue flowers that are delightfully aromatic. But wait—rub a leaf between your fingers and taste it. Is it possible? Rosemary!

Ah, so *this* is how it grows in its native climate! No wonder its name is from the Latin *ros marinus,* which translates, "dew of the sea."

Yes, rosemary can appear quite different when grown in different climates. Where the soil is sandy and well-drained, the air humid, and the sun full (such as along the Pacific Coast), rosemary is a gigantic, impressive perennial. If winter temperatures drop below 20 degrees, cut back plants and mulch well in the late fall. In even cooler areas, rosemary acts as a useful and pretty annual, rarely growing over two or three feet in height. As a potted houseplant, it remains much smaller.

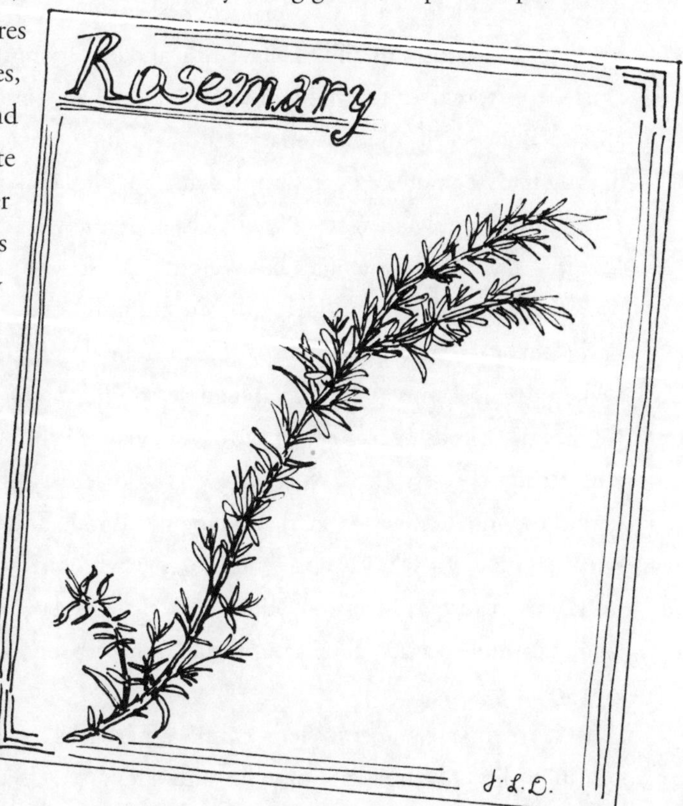

Rosemary is a sensitive plant, unable to withstand frost, cold soil, shade, wet feet, and dry air. Despite these facts, I have found it to be a surprisingly sturdy annual in my Rocky Mountain medicinal herb garden, if I work perlite (never use peat, as it's too acid for rosemary) and a bit of sand in the soil, purchase an established plant from a greenhouse, mist the leaves frequently, feed occasionally, keep in full sun, and cover at night when frost threatens. Whew! Yes, it is worth the effort.

In mild climates with humid air, this herb can easily flourish through the winter, flowering merrily during the cooler months. In climates such as mine, growing rosemary in large, well-drained pots that can be moved into the greenhouse at night (and eventually housed there for the winter) is ideal for prolonging the plant's life. Rosemary can also stand alone as a houseplant if planted in cactus-type potting soil, and given a container with sufficient drainage holes, at least six hours of sunshine, frequent misting from a spray bottle, and monthly feeding. Never overwater rosemary, as the roots will quickly rot.

Rosemary is difficult to grow from seed. Cuttings or layering work better, but buying a plant is what I consider the least discouraging way to incorporate rosemary into your garden. For harvesting and preserving, clip leaves and stem tips as needed. Store fresh rosemary in airtight containers in the refrigerator for about a week. Bunches of rosemary may be frozen whole, the leaves used as needed. To dry rosemary do not use heat. Simply hang bunches in a dark, dry, well-ventilated place until crumbly, then store in airtight containers.

After all of that, you may be wondering just why so many herb gardeners want to work with this moody plant! On the culinary scene, rosemary's powerful flavor puts it at the top of the list for seasoning strong meat flavors such as lamb, veal, and wild game. Added to Italian seasoning mixes, it is quite tasty! Baked fresh in biscuits and served with butter, the flavor is unbeatable. It also goes well with strong cheeses. The flavorful flowers of rosemary are edible, making pretty garnishes—not to mention being therapeutic as well! They are especially delightful when crystallized. Oh yes, and when rosemary blooms it is strongly attractive to honeybees, causing them to produce a particularly flavorful honey. The honey is sold at certain specialty shops and is like none other. If you can find it, try some and see!

Yes, rosemary is an excellent culinary herb. But to me the medicinal uses outshine the culinary! It is high in antioxidants, acts as an astringent, and is a powerful decongestant. Tea made from the leaves has a strong pine taste (if too strong for your liking, add a few mint leaves and a teaspoon of honey). It effectively clears stuffy heads, fights bacterial and fungal infections, eases tension, treats headaches, and is excellent for stimulating the digestive, circulatory, and nervous system functions. This tea (or an ointment containing an infusion of the leaves in olive oil and used as a topical rub) helps relieve menstrual cramps and muscle and joint pain. Or add an infusion to your bath water for a skin-healing, refreshing, invigorating start to your day (don't use before bed; lavender is the herb of choice for promoting restful sleep, while rosemary makes you more alert).

Sore throats, gum problems, and canker sores may also be treated by gargling the cooled tea, or swishing it in your mouth for three minutes as a mouthwash. According to the book *Prescription for Nutritional Healing,* rosemary tea helps detoxify the liver and has anticancer and antitumor properties. Do not exceed more than two cups per day, and for no longer than a week at a time. It is also cautioned that rosemary should not be taken by those with high blood pressure or certain other medical problems (except in culinary uses). As always, research before use!

Rosemary has excellent topical applications as well. Look at the ingredients of your favorite natural lip balm or cuticle cream, and you might see rosemary leaf oil in the list. A few drops of rosemary essential oil mixed with a drop of lavender essential oil and one cup of warm water makes a nourishing, cleansing face rinse that is good for acne and other skin disorders. Add a few drops of rosemary oil to your favorite lotion, face cream, or lip balm for a healthful improvement of skin texture and durability. Rosemary extract in shampoos and hair tonics is helpful. It prevents dandruff, revitalizes the scalp, and encourages new and healthy hair growth.

Whether in the garden, kitchen, or medicine cabinet, I think you'll agree that rosemary shines!

Tips

Add a few sprigs of rosemary to drawers and cupboards to repel moths.

In the garden, rosemary supposedly stimulates the growth of sage. They look lovely planted together too!

Rosemary planted among the rows repels cabbage moths and carrot rust flies.

OTHER MEDICINAL HERBS TO LEARN MORE ABOUT

***Licorice** (Glycyrrhiza glabra).*

This is a bushy, two- to three-foot-tall perennial with oblong, bright green leaves. The violet flowers look like tiny pea flowers, followed by reddish pods. It has thick, long roots.

Licorice has a flavor and fragrance all its own—other herbs with similar flavor and fragrance are said to "taste and smell like licorice." The roots are the part used. Licorice can be found as a flavoring in teas and candies.

With so many medicinal uses, a book could be devoted to this herb! To name a few, it cleanses the colon and fights inflammation and viral, bacterial, and parasitic infections. It improves the health of teeth and gums, reduces fever, and aids in treating menopausal symptoms.

Cautions: Shouldn't be used for more than seven days in a row. Do not use if pregnant, or if you have diabetes, glaucoma, heart disease, high blood pressure, history of stroke, extreme menstrual disorders, etc. Research well before use!

***Myrtle** (Myrtus communis).*

Do not confuse myrtle with crepe myrtle *(Lagerstroemea indica)*. Myrtle is a compact, three- to ten-foot-tall evergreen shrub. It has small, glossy, aromatic pointed leaves. In late summer, tiny, fragrant white flowers are followed by creamy white berries that ripen to blue.

Sweet, peppery taste. Pleasant aroma often used in perfumes.

Flowers make tasty garnishes; berries were once chewed by the Greeks to freshen breath; dried berries can be ground into a peppery seasoning; the oil in the sweetly fragrant leaves is for external use only, to treat bruises and painful injuries that do not break the skin. Dried leaves are good for use in potpourri and sachets. Myrtle leaves (like bay leaves) have been used in Mediterranean countries to flavor meat and game birds (the leaves are removed before serving).

Cautions: Research well before using any part of the myrtle plant.

Wintergreen *(Gaultheria procumbens).*

Also called "Checkerberry," "teaberry," and "mountain tea," you may recognize wintergreen as a flavoring in candy, root beer, and breath mints. It is a small, creeping plant with dark green, shiny leaves that have high oil content. Small white flowers are followed by brilliant scarlet berries.

Sharp, hot, peppery taste that resembles peppermint—only much stronger. Leaves, roots, and stems are used for medicinal purposes.

Wintergreen treats indigestion, skin problems, headaches, muscle pain, cold and flu symptoms, and asthma. The oil, added to a carrier oil such as almond oil, makes a good rub for rheumatism and aching muscles. Powerfully astringent.

Cautions: Undiluted essential oil irritates the skin; internal overdose is very dangerous; extended use may cause stomach and ear problems. Research well before use!

REMEMBER...

Have a healthy respect for the medicinal value of herbs. Too much of a good thing can end up causing adverse health problems. Let me repeat again: do your research and don't ignore instructions for use!

GATHERING WILD HERBS

Harvesting herbs from the wild requires accurate knowledge. Avoid all herbs growing along roadsides and fields, or wherever the soil may be polluted. Keep in mind that some wild herbs are protected and can't be harvested. Check with your local County Extension Office.

LABEL AND DATE EACH MIXTURE!

When storing herbs or making herbal preparations, list all ingredients, the recommended dose, and any cautions that apply. Add the date processed and how long it should last. This precautionary measure is vital for safe use of herbs.

CAUTION!

Keep all medicinal herbs and herbal preparations out of reach of children.

Never use washed or treated sand for gardening! The chemicals may kill your plants, but worse than that, the soil poses health risks to those who use plants grown in it for either internal or topical purposes.

PLANT CLASSIFICATION

So why are there unusual sounding Latinate words beside each common herb name? Welcome to the international system botanists have developed for classifying plants! Discussing the whole (complicated!) system would take far too much space, so I'll give a brief explanation.

Once a botanist has classified a plant down to a family (all plants therein share common characteristics), it is then narrowed down to genus (general) and species (specific) names of an individual plant. For example, French tarragon is in the Compositae family. To differentiate it from others in that family, it is given a general (genus) name, *Artemisia,* and to differentiate it from others in the same genus, it is given a specific (species) name, *dracunculus.* Since it is not the common form of *dracunculus,* but a variation, "var." is inserted, followed by the variation name, *sativa.* If a plant is a hybrid cross between two species, such as peppermint (a cross between *M. aquatica* and *M. spicata*), it will have an "x" inserted after the genus, followed by the hybrid title: *Mentha x piperita.*

While the above information doesn't cover it all, it gives a basic knowledge of how plant classification works. Imagine trying to purchase herbs (or any plant!) without the clarification of this system. It would be nearly impossible to track down the exact plant you are looking for!

Using Essential Oils

Crush the leaf and you will find how sweet it is. –Amy Carmichael

I couldn't write a book about herbs without devoting at least a few pages to essential oils! Essential oils aren't what you see (or smell) at a glance. They are the extremely valuable concentrated essences of plants. Yes, what the plant *really* is. And when I say "essential oils," I mean the 100% pure botanical extracts, not merely fragrances or synthetic reproductions (which, of course, do not contain the healthful properties of 100% pure essential oils).

The potent medicinal quality of essential oils makes them worth looking into. It's amazing what wonders are contained in one concentrated drop! The oils are also interesting (and fun!) to work with, incorporating their rich, healthful components into shampoos, lotions, muscle rubs, ointments, and teas.

Unfortunately, essential oils are sometimes associated with New Age-tainted healing practices. Aromatherapy, for example, is chiefly the use of essential oils for holistic health, a part of holism, a New Age belief system. However, "aromatherapy" has become a catch-all title for just about *any* use of essential oils (even proper use!), making it rather confusing when researching these oils. So be careful when you study the subject.[1] Ask God for wisdom and discernment to glean only the good and proper uses that He has given us in essential oils—which, by the way, are many!

Essential oils are the concentrated essences of the roots, seeds, stems, needles, leaves, bark, gums, resins, flowers, and/or fruit of a plant. Since it takes a lot of plant material to get an ounce of these precious oils, they can be rather expensive. (I consider it a worthwhile investment!) A plant must contain these oils in the first place before they can be extracted by steam distilling, cold pressing, or other procedures. For example, rosemary's aromatic leaves are high in essential oils. (Simply crush the leaves in your fingers to see/smell the rich content!) Comfrey, however, is nearly void of essential oils and therefore must be used in tinctures instead.

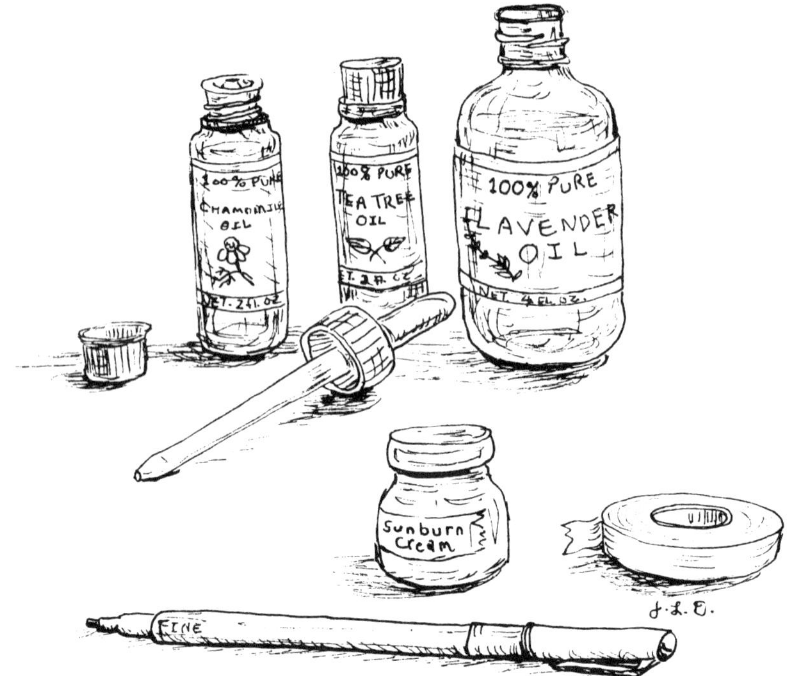

1 *The High Cost of Holistic Healing* by Dr. Nolan Byler is a good Christian-based study of holistic health practices. Published by Ridgeway Publishing (888-822-7894). It is also available through Christian Light Publications (800-776-0478).

One of the main things to remember when working with essential oils is that they are highly concentrated. As an illustration, one drop of oil is about as potent as a full cup of strongly brewed tea! I've known girls who added several drops of peppermint oil to hot water, making a drink to help ease menstrual cramps. When you consider that this one cup is equal to three very strongly brewed cups of tea, that's too much all at once! Peppermint oil is so highly potent that internal overdose can be lethal. Please use caution before making use of essential oils. Even herbs that are perfectly safe become potentially dangerous in this concentrated state. And remember, many essential oils are not safe for internal use—period. And some should not be used internally or topically during pregnancy, by people on prescription medicine, or with heart trouble, etc. Remember: do your research!

Essential oils usually need to be diluted before use. Some may be added directly to water (for foot soaks, baths, hair rinses, and so on); others need to be diluted in carrier oils such as almond oil, olive oil, coconut oil, and jojoba oil. Some do well when diluted in aloe vera gel. You may also use a glycerin base for certain essential oils. Usually oils may be directly added to shampoos, face creams, body lotions, soaps, and facial scrubs. This is a good way to begin working with essential oils, and happens to be my favorite way to use them!

Singing in the fire? Yes, God helping us, if that is the only way to get harmony out of these hard apathetic hearts, let the furnace be heated seven times hotter than before. –Mrs. C.H. Spurgeon

NOW FOR A QUICK LOOK AT SOME IMPORTANT CONSIDERATIONS:

· Only purchase quality products—don't be tempted by a low price! Usually if it's cheap, so is the content!

· Don't be surprised—100% pure essential oils have a vast range of prices, from around $4, up to about $50! The price depends on the herb, the amount of material that must be used to obtain the oil, and the process needed to procure the oil.

· Beware of imitations! It is only safe to purchase essential oils from reputable, tried-and-true companies.

· Essential oils are highly concentrated and very potent. A little goes a long way, so start out small!

· When working with undiluted essential oils, keep away from eyes, mucous membranes, etc. Wash hands after use so you won't accidentally touch sensitive areas. If small amounts of oil do get into your eyes or sensitive areas, wash with whole milk. If the amount is larger, seek medical attention immediately! ***Keep all essential oils out of reach of children!***

· Label each mixture! List all ingredients, the recommended dose, and any cautions that apply. Add the date processed and how long it should last. This precautionary measure is vital to safe use of essential oils.

· Use courtesy! Essential oils are pungent and keen in their aroma. Some people may pinch their nose against the sharp scent of tea tree oil, while others enjoy the invigorating, clean aroma. Lavender oil may soothe and calm one person's headache, but a strong whiff of it can *give* someone else a bad headache! When living under the same roof with those who can't tolerate the scent of some essential oils, be courteous. Since the initial overpowering scent usually fades quickly, sometimes a workable compromise can be found.

- Essential oils are to be used with wisdom. Don't blindly jump in and experiment! Research, research, research. Find safe uses and dosages for each essential oil you want to work with.
- When using essential oils that are new to you, dilute and test first by rubbing a small amount on the inside of your arm for three days. If a rash or irritation occurs, this essential oil is not for you!
- It is debatable if essential oils should ever be used for treating problems in small children. Don't experiment; wisely research!

TOP FIVE ESSENTIAL OIL CHOICES

These are some of my favorite oils to work with! I'll give a brief description of each.

CHAMOMILE

Dilute before use (almond oil makes a nice carrier oil). All of chamomile's excellent herbal uses are intensified in the essential oil. Use in baths, shampoos, hair rinses, massage oil, face washes, creams, body lotions, diluted in aloe vera to treat acne; it's wonderful for cleansing, anti-inflammatory, antispasmodic, and for relieving minor pain. Compresses are good for treating earache. Many more uses! Makes a delightful combination with lavender oil. Avoid if you are allergic to ragweed. Not for ingestion.

LAVENDER

Dilute before use (aloe vera works great!). This essential oil is delightfully fragrant! However, some have allergic reactions to the intensity of the scent. It's a useful, gentle antiseptic, fights bacteria, and treats fungal infection. Excellent for treating acne, burns, skin troubles, etc. Nourishing and healing when added to creams, lotions, shampoos and soaps. Sprinkle a few drops into bath water to ease muscle soreness and tension. Many more uses! Not for ingestion.

PEPPERMINT

Dilute before use (olive oil works well). Wonderful for relieving headaches, the common cold, sinus troubles, etc. It's strongly antiseptic and good for use in foot soaks (especially helpful in treating athlete's foot), baths, oral care, etc. Add to creams and lotions. Many more uses! Do not ingest, except in minimal amounts as a flavoring, in lozenges, etc.

ROSEMARY

Dilute before use (nice in almond oil). Relieves pain and has antiseptic and astringent properties. Good for circulation. Treats dandruff, hair loss, and dry, irritated skin. Helpful as a compress for relieving earaches. Many more uses! Has some cautions for those with epilepsy, asthma, etc. Do not ingest.

TEA TREE OIL

Dilute before use (aloe vera works well). Never take tea tree internally. Topically, this powerful oil is disinfectant, anti-inflammatory, antiseptic, antiviral, and so much more! It is wonderful added to aloe vera gel and used to treat rashes, acne, etc. Add to creams to treat athlete's foot. Dilute in a very small amount of olive oil or aloe vera gel and use to get rid of warts. Try a bit (a drop diluted in a drop of aloe vera gel) on insect bites and stings. Add to shampoo to treat dandruff. Many more uses! Not for ingestion.

A cup brimful of sweet water cannot spill a drop of bitter, no matter how suddenly jolted. –Unknown

ESSENTIAL OIL RECIPES

Inventing recipes is one of the most enjoyable parts of working with essential oils. I'm including just a few that I've come up with or streamlined over the years. You may have to customize!

Invigorating Foot Scrub

2 Tbsp. body wash

3 drops peppermint essential oil

2 tsp. finely ground cornmeal

Combine ingredients. Wash feet in warm water, then scrub thoroughly with Invigorating Foot Scrub. Rinse well. Pat dry and apply lotion or thick salve.

Cleansing and Refreshing Facial Scrub

1 Tbsp. mild face or body wash

1 drop tea tree essential oil or 1 drop lavender essential oil

½ tsp. finely ground cornmeal

Splash face with very warm water. Lather mixture and gently scrub face (keep away from eyes, mouth, and nostrils). Rinse thoroughly in warm water; follow with a cool rinse to close pores. Apply favorite moisturizer.

Strengthening Hand and Nail Lotion

½ c. melted cocoa butter

1 tsp. olive oil

3 drops rosemary essential oil

Whip cocoa butter until creamy. Whip in olive oil and rosemary essential oil. Store in a sealed container. Rub thoroughly into dry, cracked hands and nails before going to bed.

Dandruff-Fighter Shampoo

2 Tbsp. favorite shampoo

1 tsp. aloe vera gel

4 drops tea tree essential oil or 3 drops rosemary essential oil

Blend well. Lather into wet hair and scalp. Let sit for 30 seconds. Rinse well.

Insect Repellent Spray

This isn't for the garden; it's to keep insects away from you!

2 Tbsp. aloe vera juice

½ c. water

3 drops lemon verbena essential oil

1 drop lavender essential oil

Place in a glass spray bottle and shake well before each use. Spray on skin, but keep away from mouth, eyes, nostrils, ears, and all sensitive areas. Mixture lasts for about three months.

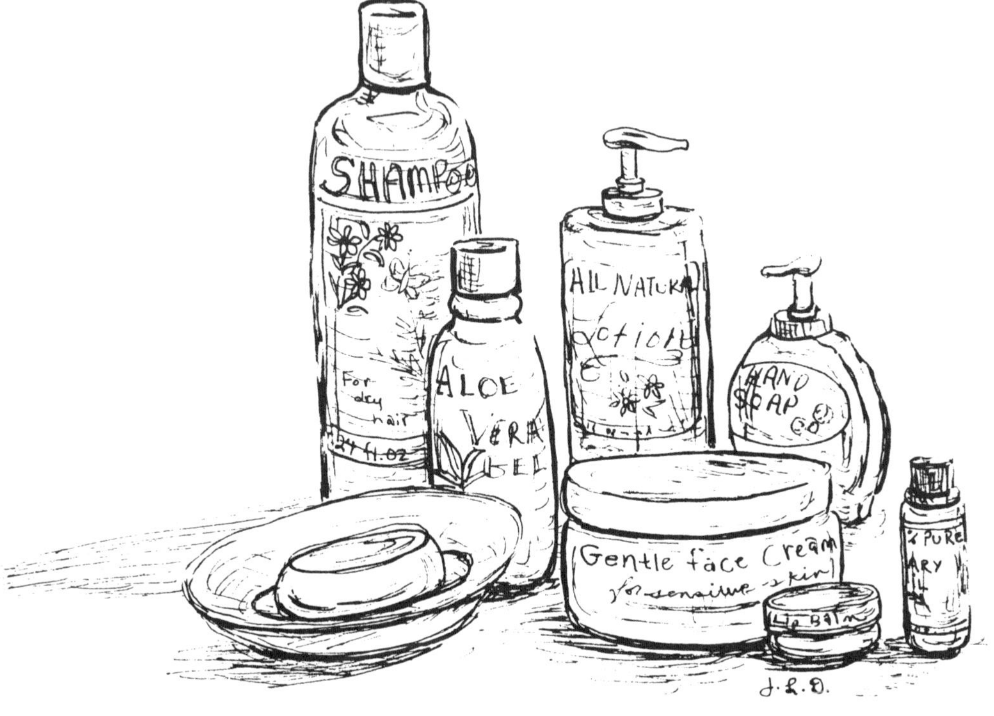

Sore Throat Soother and Astringent

½ c. warm water

6 drops tea tree essential oil

Combine and gargle (do not swallow). Repeat three times a day for one to three days.

Toothache

1 drop of clove essential oil

Apply directly to problem area to relieve pain. Don't exceed 1 drop!

Sinus-Soother Rub

1 oz. jojoba oil

1 drop basil essential oil

1 drop peppermint essential oil

1 drop eucalyptus essential oil

Combine. Rub gently on forehead and either side of the nose.

Warming Foot Soak

Suffer from icy feet? Try this!

3 drops thyme essential oil

1 Tbsp. coarse salt

8 c. hot water

Combine in a basin. Put feet in mixture and soak until water cools. Pat feet dry and immediately put on cozy socks.

If we have been learning to worship God and to trust Him, the event of a crisis will reveal that we will go to the breaking point and not break in our confidence in Him. –Oswald Chambers

The myrtle plant is small. Its flowers appear insignificant and so do its leaves. But…its leaves hold a secret. Look through them and you see numbers of small crystal balls; they look like pinpricks in the leaf. Each of these is a little vase of aromatic perfume. Crush the leaf and you will find how sweet it is.

Within each one of us is what the Bible calls "the hidden man of the heart" (1 Peter 3:4). A glance does not show it, just as a glance does not show what is in the myrtle leaves. But the moment we are carefully regarded, above all when we are tried in any way (crushed as we crush the myrtle leaf), that moment what is there is known. There is no possible way of deception. Courage or cowardice, truth or falsehood, kindness or selfishness, strength or weakness, it is known what we really are.

–Amy Carmichael

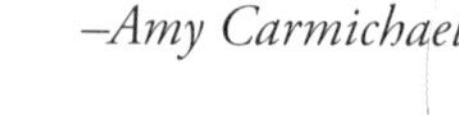

Make Your Own!

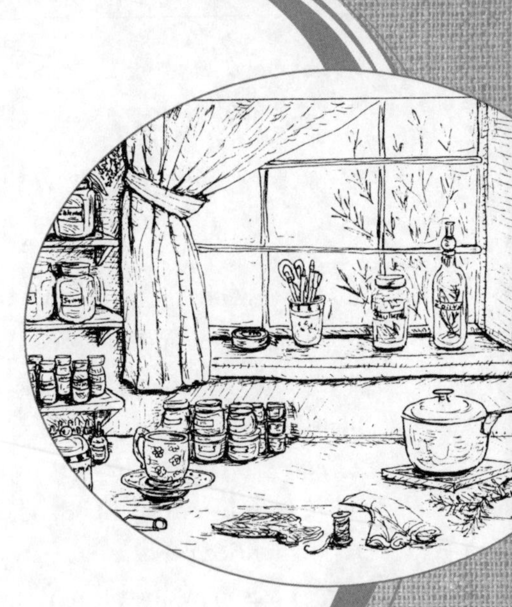

Ointment and perfume rejoice the heart (Proverbs 27:9).

THE HOW-TO FOR HERBAL PREPARATIONS

Teas, decoctions, infusions, compresses, poultices, tinctures, infused oil, infused honey, creams, ointments, balms, salves—how daunting, right? Wrong! With basic knowledge to guide you, even as a beginner you can successfully create your own herbal preparations. This chapter is to get you started; after that I believe you'll be so fascinated with the simplicity of the process and the value of the results that you'll become a confirmed home herbalist!

Once you are ready for more in-depth study, I recommend investing in a reliable guide. Your local library should have a selection of books giving detailed instructions for herbal preparations.

For now, let's discuss some of the most common herbal preparations: what they are and how to make them!

TEA

This usually means just what you think it does! And making your own is both rewarding and fun. Stainless steel tea infusers, fill-your-own tea bags, or the wonderfully convenient French press coffeemaker are excellent tea-brewing utensils.

How to: Gather the herbal parts that suit your need (usually the leaves or flowers, fresh or dried, but double the measurements for fresh). For an example, ½ teaspoon dried peppermint leaves, ½ teaspoon dried, crushed chamomile flowers, and ½ teaspoon dried lemon thyme leaves combine to make a relaxing tea that also aids digestion, promotes restful sleep, eases stress, and boosts the immune system. You may alter the measurements to suit your taste, and sometimes honey is an excellent addition!

Once you have gathered your herb(s) of choice, place in a mesh tea infuser or a tea bag, put in your favorite cup (preferably preheated), cover with 12 ounces of freshly boiled water and steep for 3 to 5 minutes. Take as needed for a tonic, immune-booster, illness-fighter, or healthful and delicious drink. If you're using a French press coffeemaker, follow the manufacturer's instructions for brewing. See tea recipes on pages 136-139.

DECOCTIONS

These are most often made from thicker parts of herbs—bark, seeds, rhizomes, berries, and/or roots. These herbal parts require simmering or boiling to extract their healing properties.

How to: A good ratio is 3 cups of fresh, cold water to ¼ cup dried herb parts or ½ cup fresh. This yields about 2 cups after simmering. Add herbs directly to cold water in a saucepan; cover and gently simmer for 15 minutes to an hour. Strain through a mesh strainer lined with cheesecloth. Gather edges of cheesecloth, fold over, and gently squeeze out the last drop of decoction through the strainer. Two cups is approximately three doses, and should be made fresh each day for internal use and refrigerated between use. Drink hot or cold. Decoctions can also be added to creams, etc. See recipes for decoctions on pages 136-139.

INFUSIONS

Infusions are medicinal-strength teas, used internally, added to bath water, or diluted and used as a hair rinse, etc. I like to keep a 4-ounce glass jar (with an eyedropper lid) filled with an infusion of one part aloe vera gel, and three parts lemon thyme-peppermint infusion. A few drops are refreshing spread over the face several times daily.

How to: Gather flowers or leafy parts of desired herbs; about 1 teaspoon dried or 2 teaspoons fresh, depending on potency needed. Place in a tea infuser or tea bag and put in a preheated cup. Bring fresh, cold water just to a boil, then pour 8 ounces over herbs. Cover cup with a saucer and allow to steep for at least 10 minutes. Press out as much liquid as possible from infuser/tea bag. Drink hot or cold. Make fresh daily.

Medicinal teas (steeped as infusions) can be purchased at health food stores. If you don't have access to the herb parts you need, purchasing ready-to-use medicinal tea bags is a simple way to start! Several excellent medicinal teas can be purchased through Nature's Warehouse (see page 225).

COMPRESSES

A compress is typically a cotton bandage soaked in herbal extracts such as infusions, decoctions, or diluted tinctures and wrapped snugly where needed. Warm compresses are helpful for ailments such as sore muscles and joints, cuts, and minor injuries; cold compresses can treat headaches and swelling.

How to: You will need strained herbal extract heated in a saucepan; a soft, clean cloth or cloth pad; plastic wrap; and a towel. For a hot compress, remove hot herbal extract from heat and soak cloth or pad in extract. Wring out (make sure it isn't too hot!) and wrap snugly or hold firmly where needed. Cover the compress with plastic wrap and a towel to retain heat. As the compress cools, dip the cloth or pad in the warm infusion and repeat. For a cold compress follow instructions above, but allow to cool before applying. See recipes for compresses on page 141.

POULTICES

Poultices are made by applying warm (or hot!) moist herbs to the skin (or spread over cotton gauze where poultice is needed), and holding snugly in place with fingers or a bandage. A very simple poultice is an herbal tea bag steeped in hot water, and then applied to problem areas (such as chamomile tea bags pressed against sore, tired eyelids). But don't stop there! Poultices are easy to make and effective for soothing aches, drawing out impurities, stimulating circulation, and so much more!

How to: It's best to use fresh herbs. Amounts will depend on the size of the affected area, so change measurements to suit. Mash or lightly run through a food processor about 2 cups of fresh herbs. Boil in a little water for about 3 to 5 minutes; press or drain excess liquid and spread herbs directly over affected area (as hot as can safely be applied). Cover with cotton strips or cloth and plastic wrap and a towel if desired. Reapply as the poultice cools. If dried herbs are all you have on hand, simply crush the herbs and mix with a bit of hot water to make a paste; apply paste between layers of cloth (to prevent skin irritation). See recipes for poultices on page 141.

TINCTURES

These are made mostly with herbs that are not fully water soluble. The main point is to draw out the full extent of medicinal properties of whatever herbs used. Vinegar, alcohol, and glycerol are solvents used for making tinctures. They draw out the healing properties of the herbs, making a potent extract. When alcohol-based tinctures are added to almost-boiling water and allowed to cool, the alcohol content will be nearly evaporated. My personal views cause me to choose only nonalcoholic tincture recipes for internal use.

Don't feel confident making tinctures all on your own? Tincture kits are available through Walnut Creek Botanicals and Bulk Herb Store (see pages 224 & 225).

How to: Put about ¼ pound crushed dried herbs or ½ pound fresh in a clean glass jar with a tightly fitting lid. Add 2½ cups glycerin or vinegar. Set the mixture in a warm place for 14 days, shaking several times daily. Or if you want to make it in 3 days instead of 14 you can use the crockpot method. Here's how: Place a clean rag in the bottom of your crockpot and put jar (filled with herbs and glycerin) on top. Fill the crockpot halfway with water and cover with lid. Turn on the lowest heat and leave it for 3 days. When it's ready, strain through cheesecloth, pressing out all liquid. Here's where a simple kitchen gadget, the potato ricer, comes in handy! It enables you to press out that last valuable drop.

Store tincture in clean, dark glass bottles. A bottle with a dropper lid is excellent since dosages are usually by drops (see recipes on pages 142-143) diluted in preparations, added to water, or taken directly depending on the tincture and the need.

INFUSED OILS

Active plant properties are extracted when infused in oil. There are two ways: hot or cold infusions. The hot method is excellent for herbs like comfrey or rosemary. The cold method is good for herbs like calendula. Medicinal herbs infused in oil are wonderful for massaging into achy joints, using in creams, ointments, etc., and much more! Cooking herbs infused in oil add flavor to marinades, sautés, etc.

How to: ***Hot infusion:*** Combine about ½ pound of fully dried herbs and 2 cups mild-tasting oil (such as sunflower oil or light olive oil) in the top of a double boiler; heat gently for about 3 hours. Pour mixture through a mesh strainer lined with cheesecloth. Gather up the cheesecloth around the herbs and press out the last drop, using your potato ricer. Pour cooled liquid into an airtight, clean, dark glass bottle.

Cold infusion: Pack thoroughly dry glass jar with about ½ pound fully dried herbs. Cover completely with oil. Place lid over the jar and set in a sunny windowsill for about 10 days, shaking several times daily. One way of checking to see if your infused oil is ready is to hold the jar up to the light. Is the oil changed to the color of the herb? Then it's ready to strain and use! Strain and bottle as with the hot infusion. See recipes for infused oils on page 144.

INFUSED HONEY

This is a wonderful way to get children to take illness-fighting or immune-boosting herbs. Adults love it too! Honey is a source for vitamins C, D, and E and B-complex. It is also gentle and soothing. Caution: do not give honey to an infant under one year of age.

How to: Warm 1 cup of honey in the top of a double boiler. Grind about 1 teaspoon dried herbs or finely chop 2 teaspoons fresh herbs; blend into honey. Warm over low heat for about 10 to 15 minutes. Strain and store in an airtight container. Excellent way to make cough and throat treatments. Honey coats the throat and allows the herbs to do their work. See recipe on page 145.

CREAMS, BALMS, SALVES, AND OINTMENTS

What's the difference? They're all oil-based mixtures, right? Yes, but they are unique! Not everyone uses the same definition for the following preparations, but here are the typical basics: Creams are more light and, well, creamy! When medicinal herbal extracts or essential oils are added, creams help the active components penetrate easily into the skin. Balms and salves are much firmer—usually beeswax is added to give the solid texture. Balms are great for healing and moisturizing dry, cracked lips. Salves are especially good for hands and feet, treating deep cracks and protecting the skin. Ointments have a pudding-like texture. They are usually based with herb-infused oils and are good for treating scrapes, cuts, bruises, etc.

How to: The process varies! Many creams have almond oil, infused oil, glycerin, and lanolin as a base. Balms commonly have more beeswax added. Salves are good with a petroleum jelly base. Ointments are excellent made from infused oil. Some nice recipes giving basic instructions can be found on pages 145-148.

EQUIPMENT FOR MAKING HERBAL PREPARATIONS

It's important to invest in equipment and utensils you will use exclusively for making herbal preparations. These can often be purchased at yard sales and thrift stores at a great bargain! Keep a list with you of the equipment you need, and begin the treasure hunt!

· Only use stainless steel, enamel, glass, or Pyrex® for pans, mixing bowls, kettles, lids, etc. Never use plastic, aluminum, or copper.

· Wooden spoons work best.

· Have a set of measuring cups and spoons specifically for working with herbs.

· A wooden cutting board.

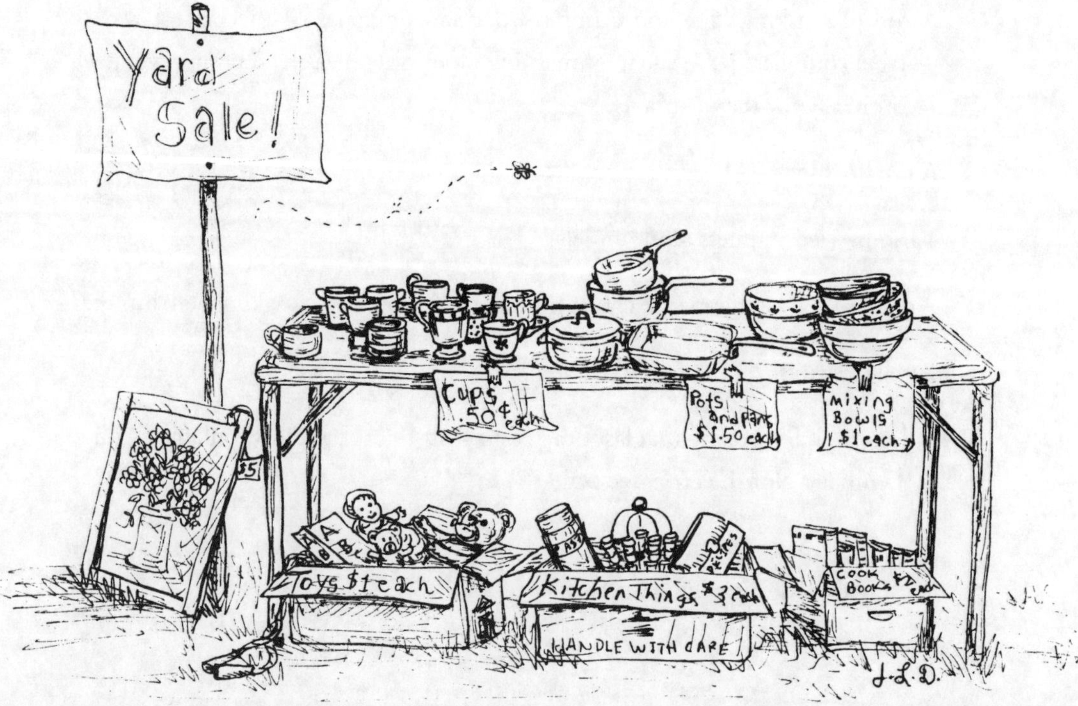

· Kitchen shears.

· Stainless steel mesh strainers/sieves.

· Canning jars.

· 1 and 2 ounce glass bottles (best if amber or cobalt colored to protect the content from too much light exposure), preferably with glass eyedropper lids, or a dropper insert under the lid. I save the empty bottles from the essential oils I buy; washed and dried, these are perfect for storing small amounts of tinctures, diluted essential oils, etc.

· Airtight glass canisters for storing bulk dried herbs.

· Small airtight glass containers with plastic inserts (which make sprinkling easy) under the lid. These are great for storing dried herbs. Keep your eyes open at yard sales! I've found many spice racks with empty spice jars—usually at giveaway prices. I guess some folks don't realize you can reuse these! Simply wash well in hot, soapy water with a drop of bleach to sanitize. Rinse well and dry thoroughly before filling.

· A roll of masking tape and a fine-tip permanent marker—the perfect way to label your glass jars! A strip of masking tape goes on easily, stays put, yet peels off nicely for the next label.

· A quality blender.

· Various-sized stainless steel funnels.

· A good supply of fine-weave cheesecloth for straining, or for making herb bundles.

· Kitchen string.

· Potato ricer, for getting that last drop from your tinctures, etc. (available through Lehman's Non-Electric; see page 224).

· French press coffeemaker—nice and convenient for teas and infusions (also available through Lehman's; see page 224).

Using Herbs for Healing

Recipes for making your own herbal remedies

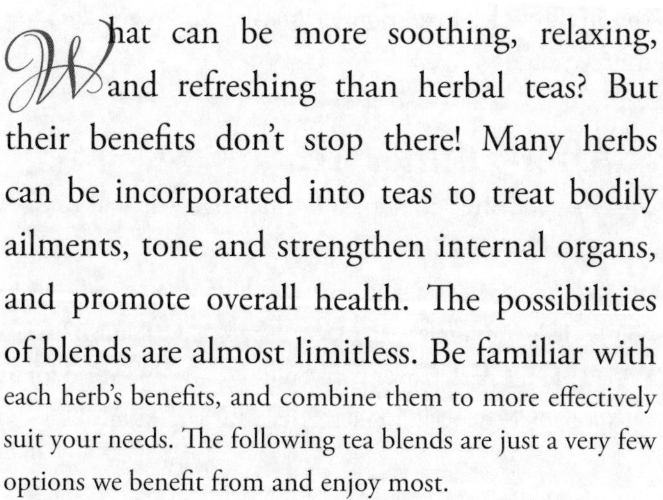

What can be more soothing, relaxing, and refreshing than herbal teas? But their benefits don't stop there! Many herbs can be incorporated into teas to treat bodily ailments, tone and strengthen internal organs, and promote overall health. The possibilities of blends are almost limitless. Be familiar with each herb's benefits, and combine them to more effectively suit your needs. The following tea blends are just a very few options we benefit from and enjoy most.

Herbs may be steeped into teas either fresh or dried. One teaspoon dried herbs is usually equal to 1 tablespoon fresh.

Teas, Decoctions, & Infusions

Pick-Me-Up Tea

Want a refreshing, cooling tea that is also helpful in relieving indigestion? Harvest a few leaves from lemon verbena, lemongrass, and lemon thyme. Chop herbs (the result should be about 1 tablespoon herbs) and place in a tea infuser. Cover with boiling water and steep for 3 to 5 minutes. Sweeten with honey if desired; serve hot and enjoy! Or serve over ice to bring down body temperature after overexertion.

Good-for-You Tea

A delicious, nutritious tea my sister came up with includes the leaves of peppermint, lemon thyme, and lime basil. Sometimes we add a bag of black tea for a full, rich, antioxidant-rich cup. This healthful tea is an immune booster, and is excellent for treating headaches, taut nerves, and indigestion.

After-Dinner Tea

Dried coriander seed makes a good after-dinner tea for digestive help and to ease bloating. This combination is also helpful for clearing the complexion if taken daily for a week. For one 8-ounce power-packed cup, combine in a tea infuser: 6 dried seeds and ½ teaspoon dried lemongrass (slightly crushed), 2 fresh mint leaves (torn), and ¼ teaspoon dried orange peel. Cover with boiling water and steep for 5 to 7 minutes (covered). Especially beneficial if taken after your largest meal.

Friendships are nourished over a pot of tea. –Unknown

Mint Medley

What can beat peppermint tea? Some say it's invigorating, some call it relaxing, and most agree that it is deliciously refreshing and calming. Even the scent soothes the nerves! Peppermint tea is known to relieve sinus congestion and ease indigestion, tension headaches, and nerves. It builds the immune system and helps ward off the common cold. Wonderful served hot or cold. Place 2 tablespoons fresh (chopped) leaves or 2 teaspoons dried in a tea infuser. Cover with 8 ounces of freshly boiled water. Steep for 3 minutes. Add honey if desired. It's also fun to add different mint flavors! Try apple mint, orange mint, or pineapple mint for great variation. Yum!

Snooze Tea

Need a bedtime tea? Combine ¼ teaspoon dried (crushed) lemongrass, ¼ teaspoon dried peppermint, ¼ teaspoon dried lemon balm, and ¼ teaspoon dried chamomile. Cover with 8 ounces freshly boiled water and steep for 3 minutes. Sweeten with honey if desired. Ahhh...relaxing!

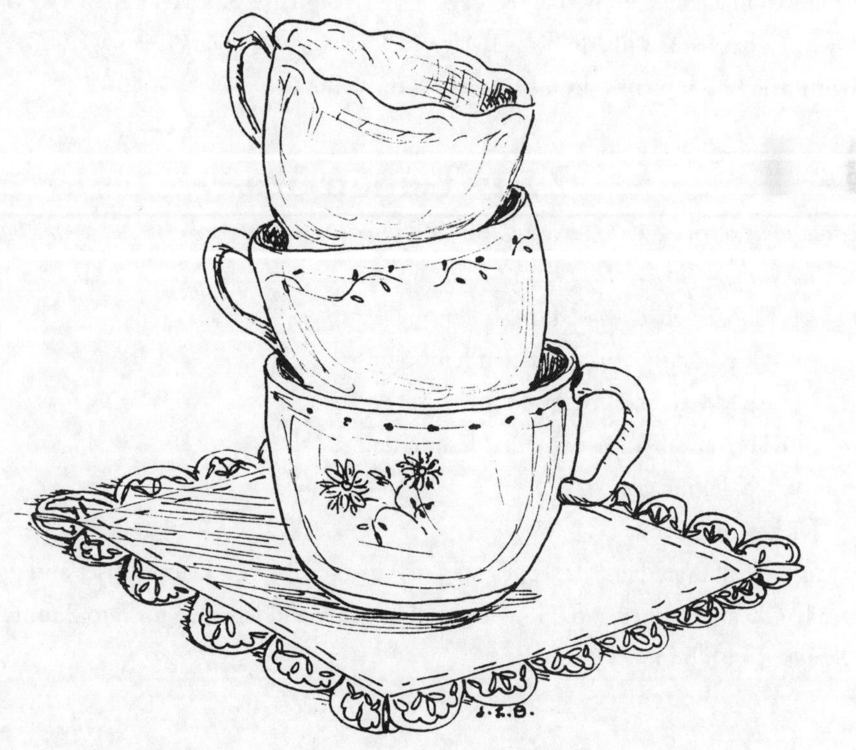

Cough Tea

Can't beat that annoying cough? Make a 10-minute decoction of ½ teaspoon dried licorice root and ½ teaspoon freshly grated gingerroot in ¾ cup water. Strain. Meanwhile, in a large mug pour 1 cup of freshly boiled water over a tea bag filled with dried red clover tops. Cover and steep for 5 minutes. Add about ½ cup of the hot licorice/ginger decoction and sweeten with honey. See if that doesn't do the trick!

Get-Well Tea

Here's a tasty tea that builds the immune system and fights the common cold: Combine in a tea infuser dried peppermint leaves, echinacea root, rose hips, and lemon thyme. Steep in boiling water for 5 minutes. Sweeten with honey. Delicious!

Tea as Gifts

Want to make custom herbal tea bags to have on hand or give as gifts? Fill-your-own tea bags are available from Backyard Herbs and Flowers (see page 223). Fill with dried herb blends, iron shut, label, and enjoy!

Zesty Lemon Tea

Absolutely bursting with lemon flavor and vitamin C, this makes a wonderful hot or cold beverage—any time of day!

1 Tbsp. finely chopped, fresh lemongrass or
  1 tsp. gently crushed, dried lemongrass
½ tsp. dried, crushed rose hips
½ Tbsp. fresh or ½ tsp. dried lemon balm
¼ tsp. lemon zest
1 bag of green tea

Combine all ingredients (except green tea) in a tea infuser. Place infuser and green tea bag in an 8-ounce cup. Fill with boiling water and let steep for 5 to 7 minutes. Sweeten with honey if desired.

Sniffle-Stopping Tea

As soon as you feel a cold coming on, brew a steaming cup of this immune-boosting tea.

½ tsp. dried, crushed echinacea root

½ tsp. dried mint leaves

½ tsp. dried, crushed lemongrass

Combine herbs in a tea infuser. Cover with 8 ounces of freshly boiled water. Cover and steep for 8 to 10 minutes. Sweeten with honey. Take twice daily. Do not consume for more than 5 to 7 days in a row. This tea is also good for treating urinary tract infections.

Mullein-Petal Tea

This tea should be taken in small doses, not exceeding 2 cups a day for 5 days in a row. It is excellent for relieving coughs and hoarseness. Best taken before bedtime or in the morning.

1 Tbsp. fresh mullein flower petals

8 ounces boiling water

1 tsp. honey

Steep petals in water until the water is golden. Remove petals and stir in honey. Drink slowly.

Sore-Throat Rescue

1 tsp. dried, ground echinacea root

1 tsp. dried, ground licorice root

1 tsp. dried lemon balm leaf

Combine in a saucepan and simmer in 2 cups of water for about 10 minutes. Remove from heat; cover and steep for 10 minutes more. Strain out plant material, squeezing to extract all liquid. Allow to cool and store in the refrigerator for up to a week. Gargle 1 to 2 Tbsp. liquid to ease sore throat, or blend ½ cup honey with ¼ cup liquid and take by the Tbsp. to ease sore throat and boost the immune system.

Aloe Vera Morning Smoothie

This tasty drink mixture is high in vitamin C and fortifies the immune system. Vanilla yogurt lightly sweetens the blend, while imparting "friendly" bacteria and digestive-boosting properties. Aloe vera is good for lowering cholesterol, improving circulation in the lower extremities, soothing and healing stomach and esophageal irritation, and acting as a mild laxative. The addition of cranberry juice is excellent for the bladder, urinary tract, kidneys, and skin health. Both aloe vera and cranberries fight "unfriendly" bacteria and help ward off infection. Do not use for more than 5 to 7 days without a break. Avoid during pregnancy.

Fill an ice cube tray with cranberry juice; freeze. In a blender, place ½ cup aloe vera juice and ½ cup vanilla yogurt. Add 6 cranberry juice ice cubes. Blend until smooth. Yield: 2 servings. Note: If this mixture is too tart for your taste buds, try a cranberry juice that has been combined with the natural sweetness of apple juice or mixed berries.

Cut, Scratch, and Scrape Rescue

1 cup water

¼ cup fresh rosemary or 1½ Tbsp. dried

1 Tbsp. commercially prepared witch hazel

Simmer rosemary in water for 10 minutes; remove from heat, cover, and steep for 10 minutes more. Strain out leaves. Stir in witch hazel. Store in the refrigerator for up to 3 months. Saturate a sterile cotton pad with mixture and dab gently on problem area. Repeat up to 3 times a day for a week.

I ran away from a thousand things waiting to be done and stole a little visit with a friend. –Laura Ingalls Wilder

Poultices & Compresses

Bruise-Healing Poultice

⅓ cup chopped, fresh mullein leaves

⅔ cup water

In a saucepan, simmer leaves for about 20 minutes. Spoon warm (not hot!) mixture onto thin cotton and secure over bruised area.

Plantain Poultice

The healing, antibiotic, and antiseptic properties of plantain leaves make them excellent treatment for blisters, slight wounds, and sores. They also take the pain out of insect stings and bites.

1 cup water

½ cup fresh plantain leaves, torn

¼ cup fresh calendula petals

In a saucepan, bring water to a boil; remove from heat. Stir in herbs, cover, and steep for 5 minutes. Scoop out warm, wet herbs and place on problem area. Wrap with gauze and leave on until cold. Allow area to air dry. Repeat 3 times a day. The liquid from the herbs may also be dabbed onto the problem area.

Healing Compress

2 cups water

1 Tbsp. ground dried plantain leaves

½ Tbsp. ground dried echinacea root

Boil water; pour over herbs. Cover and steep for 15 minutes. Strain and cool to warm temperature. Dip soft, clean cloth into infusion and lightly wring out. Apply to minor wounds or infections. Secure in place and leave on until cloth is cold. Repeat 3 to 5 times a day.

Tinctures

The Immune Booster

2 cups echinacea
1 cup echinacea root
1 cup stinging nettle leaves
1 cup peppermint leaves
vegetable glycerin
½ cup boiling water

Mix the dry herbs together. Fill a quart jar ⅓ full with your herb mixture. Store the rest in a glass jar or ziplock bag for later use. Be sure to label it and keep instructions with the mix for your convenience. After filling the quart jar ⅓ full, pour ½ cup boiling water on the dry herbs then fill the jar with glycerin to within 1 inch from top. Stir the gooey mixture well, then cap with screw-on lid. Place clean rag in bottom of crockpot and put jar on top. Fill crockpot halfway with water and cover with lid. Turn to lowest heat and leave for 3 days. Don't let the crock get too low on water. After 3 days strain through clean cloth, discard herbs, and store the liquid tincture in a labeled glass jar. Keep in pantry or other cool, dark place. Adult dosage: ½–1 Tbsp. hourly. Children ages 1–12 can be given 2 droppers hourly and children under 1 year ½ dropper hourly.

Super Tonic

¼ cup garlic

¼ cup onion

¼ cup horseradish

¼ cup gingerroot

¼ cup cayenne pepper

unpasteurized apple cider vinegar

Peel garlic, onion, horseradish, and gingerroot. Chop in blender with cayenne pepper, adding vinegar if necessary to facilitate the chopping process. Pour into quart jar and fill to within 1 inch of top with apple cider vinegar. Stir well and cover with plastic lid if possible (prevents corrosion) or just use regular canning lid with screw-on band. Let set for 3 weeks, then strain. Save liquid in a labeled glass jar discarding the rest. Adult dosage when ill is 1 Tbsp. hourly. Can be diluted and sweetened for children. It is handy to put tape on jar with the date written on when it will be ready. Good to use as a gargle for sore throat.

Outside there's ice on the stark, bare trees
And snow on the ground—but inside, there's me
Up near the fire with a cup in hand;
I heed not the chill of the winter-land.
I've a steaming cup of peppermint tea
(It was growing once in the garden, you see,
When the days were long and the sun shone warm,
And the grass was green, and the trees unshorn),
And last summer's taste, so it seems to me,
Is found in a cup of peppermint tea.
–J.L.D.

Infused Oils & Honey

Calendula Infused Oil

1 sterilized glass pint jar (Make sure it's thoroughly dry! Any moisture spoils the oil.)
⅔ cup thoroughly dried calendula petals
enough olive oil to cover dried petals and nearly fill the jar

Place dried calendula in the jar. Cover with olive oil. Place a coffee filter over the top and secure with a rubber band. Set on a sunny windowsill or porch rail for about a week. Strain out calendula petals. Place strained oil into clean glass bottles; label and date. Lasts for about 3 months if stored in a cool, dry, dark place.

Or, for a quicker variation: Place ⅔ cup dried petals and 2 cups olive oil in the top of a double boiler. Simmer very gently for about an hour. Cool mixture; strain out the petals. Place in clean glass jars; label and date. Lasts for about 3 months if stored in a cool, dry, dark place.

Both recipes are not for internal use. They are wonderful for treating skin troubles—a dab is so soothing! May be added to creams and lotions.

Mullein Infused Oil

Mullein infused oil is good for treating earaches and many skin troubles. It reduces inflammation and numbs pain, plus makes a good base for first-aid ointments.

⅓ cup dried, chopped mullein leaves
2 cups olive oil

In the top of a double boiler, place olive oil and mullein leaves. Simmer gently for about an hour. Cool and strain carefully. Place in clean glass jars; label and date. Lasts for about 3 months in a cool, dry, dark place.

Throat-Soother Infused Honey

1 quart wildflower honey

¼ cup dried lemongrass, crushed, or ½ cup fresh and finely chopped

In the top of a double boiler, warm honey. Add lemongrass and warm for about 15 minutes. Strain; pour into a canning jar and cover tightly with lid. Label jar. Keeps for about 6 months if stored in a cool, dark place. Take a teaspoonful up to 5 times a day to soothe and heal a sore throat.

Creams, Balms, Salves, & Ointments

Calendula Comfort Cream

This rich cream comforts dry, rough, sore, or chapped skin and heals small cuts. And it smells good too!

½ Tbsp. beeswax

1 Tbsp. cocoa butter

½ Tbsp. almond oil

1 tsp. glycerin

1½ tsp. calendula oil (see page 144 for *Calendula Infused Oil* recipe)

3 drops chamomile essential oil

3 drops rose essential oil

Melt beeswax; blend in cocoa butter. Warm almond oil and stir in glycerin; add calendula oil and essential oils. Stir into beeswax mixture. Place in clean jars and label.

Lemon Balm

Make a hot or cold infusion of olive oil and lemon balm. Gently heat 1 cup of the oil. In a separate pan, gently melt ½ ounce of beeswax. Blend into warm oil. Add more beeswax to reach desired consistency.

Comfrey Salve

Make a hot infusion of comfrey and olive oil. Gently heat 1 cup of infused oil. In a separate saucepan, gently melt 1 ounce of beeswax. Blend into warm oil. Cool and place in a glass or tin container. Lasts for about 1 year. This salve is excellent for preventing scars!

Salve for Cracked, Dry Skin

½ cup petroleum jelly
1 Tbsp. fresh comfrey, finely chopped
2 tsp. dried chamomile flowers, crushed
2 drops tea tree essential oil

In a double boiler, gently melt petroleum jelly; stir in comfrey and chamomile. Remove from heat (gently reheating whenever mixture begins to cool), cover, and let infuse for 45 minutes. Add tea tree oil. Strain through a mesh strainer into a glass jar or tin. Cool completely; cover with lid.

Replenishing Body Lotion

⅔ cup olive oil
1 tsp. wheat germ
¼ cup fresh lavender (leaves and flowers)
¼ cup fresh chamomile flowers
½ cup mild body lotion
1 tsp. honey

In the top of a double boiler, add olive oil, wheat germ, and herbs. Simmer gently for 30 minutes. Remove from heat, strain well, and combine oil with remaining ingredients in a clean jar with a lid. Shake until creamy. Apply as often as desired.

Antiseptic Wash for Sensitive Skin

This is effective for clearing up acne. It speeds cell replacement while gently cleansing and nourishing skin.

1 cup water

¼ cup fresh lavender (flowers and leaves)

Place in a saucepan, cover, and gently simmer for 20 minutes. Remove from heat, cover and let steep for 20 minutes more. Cool and strain. Place infusion in a clean glass jar; label and date. Dilute in warm water (¼ cup to 1 cup water) and splash over face after washing. Pat dry and follow with favorite moisturizer. Use within 5 to 7 days.

Lavender Ointment

Make a hot infused oil using lavender leaves and flowers. This will be the base of your salve (see page 131 for instructions on making hot oil infusions). In a separate saucepan, gently melt ½ ounce of cocoa butter. Blend with 1 cup warm infused lavender oil. Allow to cool completely. Is it too thin? Warm gently and add a small chip of melted beeswax. Too thick? A drop or two more of the oil should help. When completely cool, store in small glass jars or 4-ounce tin cans made for salves, etc. Lasts for about a year.

Want to turn your Lavender Ointment into a salve or balm? Here's how! Simply add more beeswax to reach the consistency you want.

Healing After-Sunburn Lotion

⅔ cup aloe vera gel

2 capsules vitamin E, split and the contents squeezed out

1 drop tea tree oil

2 drops chamomile oil

2 Tbsp. mild face cream

Place all ingredients in a clean 4-ounce jar with a lid; shake until smooth. Gently apply directly on sunburn at least 3 times a day. Good for treating other minor skin irritations as well.

Soother Salve

2 oz. yarrow

2 oz. comfrey

½ tsp. vitamin E (contents of 2–500 IU capsules)

1 pint olive oil

1¼ oz. beeswax

Combine herbs and oil in small kettle. Heat gently (do not boil) for 1 hour, stirring occasionally. Strain and discard herbs. Pour liquid back into kettle; add beeswax and vitamin E until melted. Immediately pour into shallow tins or small glass jars. Let cool before covering.

Dill Rub for Achy Muscles

2 Tbsp. minced dill

1 Tbsp. olive oil

1 Tbsp. avocado oil

Blend dill and oils in a glass jar. Set in a sunny windowsill for 24 hours. Press through a cheesecloth-lined strainer into a clean glass jar with a lid; label and date (lasts for about 1 month). Massage into achy muscles when needed.

Come, ye thankful people, come—
Raise the song of harvest home:
All is safely gathered in
Ere the winter storms begin.
God, our Maker, doth provide
For our wants to be supplied:
Come to God's own temple, come—
Raise the song of harvest home.
–Henry Alford

Facial & Whole Body Rinses

Echinacea Facial Rinse

This calming, anesthetic rinse promotes healing and reduces the painful irritation of many skin disorders, including burns, eczema, acne, and most rashes.

In a saucepan, combine 1 tsp. dried, crushed echinacea root and 2 cups water. Bring to a boil; lower heat and simmer, covered, for 10 minutes. Remove from heat; strain out root particles. Cool infusion and splash over infected areas after gently washing. Pat dry; apply favorite moisturizer.

Parsley Facial Rinse

This refreshing rinse is a nice remedy for oily skin.

Place several sprigs of fresh parsley, or 1 Tbsp. dried, in a dish. Pour 2 cups boiling water over the leaves. Cover and let steep for 20 minutes. Strain out leaves. Use the infusion as a cleansing facial rinse after washing. Follow with cool water; pat dry and apply favorite moisturizer.

Lemongrass Facial Wash

This deliciously scented herb has natural cleansing properties and is rich in vitamin A. Use this wash to clear the skin and improve its texture. You may also skip the liquid face wash ingredient and simply dilute the infusion in warm water for a hair rinse to treat oily hair.

¼ cup water

1 Tbsp. finely chopped fresh lemongrass

In a saucepan, bring water and lemongrass to a boil; simmer for 2 minutes. Remove from heat and cover; steep for 15 minutes. Strain out plant material; reserve liquid. Add infusion to 1 cup of gentle liquid face wash (will keep for about 3 to 4 weeks). Rinse skin with very warm water; gently apply face wash mixture; rinse well with warm water and follow with cool water. Apply favorite moisturizer. Gentle enough to be used daily.

Skin-Nourishing Soap

Rosemary nourishes the skin and improves texture and durability. It's also gently cleansing.

2 cups bar soap pieces

¼ cup fresh rosemary, gently bruised

1 cup water

Collect stray bits of end-of-the-bar soap until you have about 2 cups' worth. Place in a saucepan reserved for such purposes. In another pan with a lid, simmer water and rosemary over low heat for 30 minutes. Strain out plant material and pour hot liquid over soap. Gently heat and stir until mushy. When the mixture is cool enough to handle, shape into balls or press into soap molds. Allow to thoroughly dry for a week. Store in an airtight jar.

Strengthening Hair Rinse

1 tsp. dried thyme

½ tsp. dried mint leaves

½ tsp. dried rosemary leaves

Gently crush herbs. Cover with 2 cups boiling water and steep for 20 minutes. Strain and squeeze out every drop from herbs. Add 1 Tbsp. cider vinegar to the water and 1 cup warm water. Wash hair as usual, followed by the rinse mixture. Follow with a cool rinse.

Natural Cleanser and Deodorant

Infuse ⅛ cup dried lovage leaves and roots along with ¼ cup dried sage leaves in 1 cup water. Strain. Add several drops of lavender essential oil to liquid. Splash underarms after a bath.

Sleepy-Time Bath

Here's a muscle-relaxing, tension-taming mixture that promotes restful sleep while nourishing, conditioning, and cleansing the skin.

In a saucepan, combine 2 cups water and ¼ cup each of dried lavender and dried chamomile. Simmer for 10 minutes; remove from heat, cover, and steep for 10 minutes more. Strain out plant material. Pour liquid into bath water.

Healing, Softening Bath for Problem Skin

Do you suffer from dry, cracked skin that is irritated and uncomfortable? This bath, repeated at least twice a week, might be the cure. Avoid if pregnant.

In a saucepan, combine 4 cups water, 1 cup fresh, chopped comfrey leaves, and 1 Tbsp. fresh, chopped roots (optional). Simmer gently for about 20 minutes; remove from heat and cover. Allow to steep for 20 minutes. Strain out plant particles carefully. Pour liquid into a clean glass jar and keep in the refrigerator for up to a month. Add ½ cup to bath water when desired. This is also a good infusion to add to skin creams and lotions.

Relaxing, Healing Herbal Bedtime Bath

2 Tbsp. dried chamomile
2 Tbsp. dried lavender
1 Tbsp. dried comfrey leaves
3 cups water

In a saucepan, combine herbs and water. Simmer on low for about 5 minutes. Remove from heat, cover, and let stand for 5 more minutes. Strain out herbs and pour liquid into bath water. Eases tension, relaxes muscles, and benefits the skin.

Sunburn-Reliever Water

Here's a way to soothe the pain from a sunburn, while healing and nourishing the skin. May be added directly to bath water, splashed on affected areas, or used as a scalp rinse.

2 Tbsp. dried chamomile
1 Tbsp. dried comfrey (root and leaves)
1 tsp. crushed fennel seeds
2 cups water

In a saucepan, add herbs and water. Simmer on low for 5 minutes. Remove from heat, cover, and let stand for 5 more minutes. Strain out herbs. Cool completely. Dilute with cool water and use as needed.

Skin-Calming Splash

½ cup aloe vera gel
3 Tbsp. witch hazel
1 Tbsp. lemon juice
2 drops lavender oil

Place in a 6-ounce bottle with a tight-fitting lid and shake well. Apply often to problem skin to cleanse, calm, and nourish. Store in a cool, dark place. Lasts for up to 6 months.

Gentle Bath Infusion

This bath infusion is simple!

Gather 1 Tbsp. each of dried chamomile, lavender, and rosemary; infuse in 2 cups hot water. Strain, cool completely, then add ½ tsp. salt, 1 tsp. cider vinegar, 2 tsp. aloe vera gel, and 2 drops lavender essential oil or 1 drop chamomile essential oil. Add to bath when running the water. Excellent for sensitive skin!

Rejuvenating Bay Leaf Bath for Tired Toes

3 Tbsp. dried bay leaf

1 Tbsp. coarse salt

Place in a large basin. Pour in 6 cups boiling water. Cover and steep until cool enough to place your feet in the basin. Get a good book, sit in a comfy chair, and soak your feet for 10 minutes.

Cleansing, Nourishing Bath Water

This is a beneficial addition to your bath, both cleansing and nourishing for the skin, leaving it fresh and soft.

2 Tbsp. dried bay leaves

1 Tbsp. dried lavender flowers and leaves

1 Tbsp. finely ground oatmeal

1 Tbsp. finely ground bran

4 cups water

Place in a saucepan. Simmer for about 20 minutes, stirring occasionally. Strain. Pour liquid into bath water.

Fun Recipes to Try

Respiratory Soother Drops

3½ lb. brown sugar

3 cups water

2 oz. dried horehound

In a saucepan, bring water and horehound to a boil. Remove from heat, cover, and let steep for 20 minutes. Strain leaves, squeezing out excess to get fullest flavor. Add brown sugar and cook and stir over low heat until the hard ball stage (250°). Pour into a greased dish and allow to cool. Grease hands and shape candy into balls; flatten to form disks. Let cool completely and store in an airtight container in the refrigerator for about 3 to 5 days.

Crystallized Horehound Leaves

fresh horehound leaves
egg white
sugar

Whisk egg white with a fork until nearly foaming. Hold leaf by stalk and dip into egg white to completely coat. Dip in sugar, turning to coat. Lay on a wax paper-covered baking sheet. Repeat with remaining leaves. Heat oven to 200°; turn it off. Place baking sheet on the middle rack until leaves are brittle. Cool completely. Store in an airtight container. These are very strong tasting and super good! They are helpful for treating coughs and respiratory troubles.

Comfrey Fertilizer

Comfrey leaves are bursting with healthful substances and loaded with protein. They especially benefit potatoes and tomatoes due to the high potash content they impart into the soil. Try this fertilizer—I think you'll appreciate the results!

Fill a large kettle with 6 cups water; add about 2 cups of fresh, torn comfrey leaves. Stir to mix. Cover and simmer for about 30 minutes, stirring occasionally. Remove from heat and let steep for about 15 minutes. Strain out leaves; dilute liquid equally (1 cup water to 1 cup liquid) and pour into soil around plants.

Moth Repellent Blend

This combination is wonderfully fragrant—while working effectively to keep moths at bay! Tuck sachets into chests, linen cabinets, and dresser drawers. Hang some in your closets too!

1 cup dried lavender leaves and flowers
⅔ cup dried rosemary
½ cup dried mint
½ cup dried thyme
⅓ cup dried tansy

Mix together and place about ¼ cup into a cotton sachet bag (recipe will fill about 12 bags). Crush the bags gently (to release the fragrance of the herbs) before tucking them away.

Cooking with Herbs

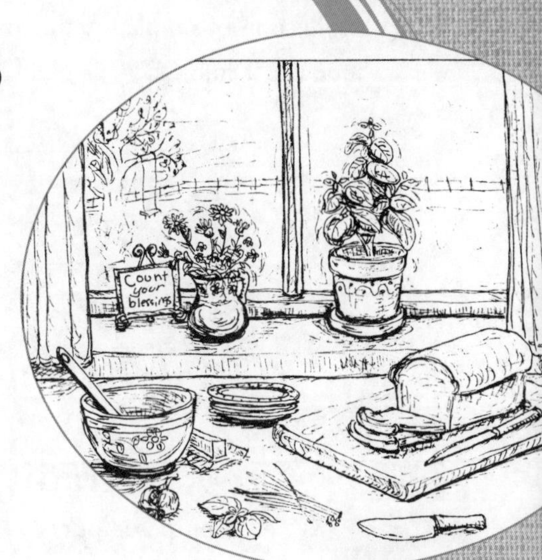

Better is a dinner of herbs where love is, than a stalled [fatted] ox and hatred therewith (Proverbs 15:17).

WELCOME TO MY HERB KITCHEN

As I've mentioned over and over, herb gardening has many benefits. For example, gathering herbs in the cool of a late summer morning. What can beat *that* for recreation?! And I simply love being surrounded by the beauty of varied tones and textures of green, and those delicate little blossoms in rainbow hues. But for me, this enjoyment is followed closely by one of my favorite of life's simple pleasures: incorporating herbs into recipes. Compiling recipes for the use of herbs was a mind-boggling feat. It actually took willpower to narrow down the vast assortment of choices! The result is a collection of simple, useful, and delicious recipes and tips that I enjoy most. I hope you'll enjoy them as well!

Herb Breads, Biscuits, & Scones

Traditional Rye Bread

4-5 c. all-purpose flour
2½ tsp. active dry yeast
2 c. warm water
¼ c. packed brown sugar
1 Tbsp. molasses
2 Tbsp. olive oil
1¼ tsp. salt
1½ c. rye flour
1 heaping Tbsp. caraway seeds

Mix 3 cups all-purpose flour and yeast. In a separate mixing bowl combine warm water, brown sugar, molasses, oil, and salt. Beat into dry mixture until smooth, for about 1 minute. Add rye flour, caraway seeds, and enough all-purpose flour to make a firm dough. Turn onto a floured surface and knead for 5 minutes. Place in a greased bowl, turning once to grease top. Cover and let rise in a warm place for about an hour. Punch dough down and divide in half. Grease baking sheet. Shape each half of dough into a ball, tucking the edges under and placing on the baking sheet. Flatten each loaf until it is 6" around. Score tops with a sharp knife. Cover and let rise for about 30 minutes. Preheat oven to 375°. Bake loaves for 30-35 minutes. Cool on wire racks. Delicious served warm topped with slices of cheddar cheese and alfalfa sprouts. Or simply spread with butter. Yum!

Garlic and Cheese Herb Bread

1 large loaf French or sourdough bread, split

2 garlic cloves, peeled and crushed

1 Tbsp. chopped fresh parsley

1 tsp. finely chopped fresh thyme

¼ c. snipped fresh garlic leaves or chives

12 tsp. softened butter

¼ c. mayonnaise

1 c. shredded mozzarella cheese

Split loaf in half, placing both halves on a baking sheet, cut side up. Mix all other ingredients except cheese. Spread on bread halves; sprinkle with cheese. Preheat oven to 350° and bake until cheese is melted and topping is bubbly, about 10-15 minutes.

First butter, then:
The tang of chives,
A basil hint;
A garlic touch
And I'm content
To chop and mix
This yummy spread
And serve it with
A loaf of bread!
–J.L.D.

Chicory Bread

This dark, nutritious bread has a mild chicory flavor that complements the nutty taste of whole wheat.

3½ c. all-purpose flour
2½ tsp. active dry yeast
1¾ c. water
⅓ c. packed brown sugar
3 Tbsp. olive oil
1 tsp. salt
3 Tbsp. dried, ground chicory root
2 c. whole wheat flour

In a large bowl, combine yeast with 2 cups all-purpose flour; set aside. In a medium saucepan heat water, brown sugar, oil, and salt until warm. Beat into flour mixture for about 1 minute. In a separate bowl, mix together whole wheat flour and dried chicory root. Add to dough mixture. Mix in as much remaining all-purpose flour as possible. Turn onto a floured surface and knead for 5 minutes. Place in a greased bowl, turning once to grease top. Cover and let rise in a warm place for about 1 hour. Punch dough down. Divide in half and shape into 2 loaves. Place in greased bread pans, cover, and let rise for about half an hour. Preheat oven to 375°. Bake bread for 35-40 minutes, or until it sounds hollow when tapped. Cool for at least 10 minutes before slicing.

Lemony-Sweet Quick Bread

¾ c. milk

1 c. plus 2 Tbsp. fresh lemon balm (divided)

1 Tbsp. fresh lemon thyme

½ c. butter, softened

1 c. sugar

2 eggs

2¼ c. all-purpose flour

1½ tsp. baking powder

¼ tsp. salt

Spread:

¼ c. butter, softened

1 tsp. grated lemon zest

2 Tbsp. honey

Preheat oven to 325°. Gently crush herbs (except 2 Tbsp. lemon balm) and place in a saucepan. Cover with milk. Bring to a boil, then immediately remove from heat and cover. When cool, strain out herbs and reserve infused milk. Combine butter, sugar, and eggs, beating well. In a separate bowl, combine flour, baking powder, and salt. Add to butter mixture alternately with infused milk. Add 2 Tbsp. lemon balm to batter. Pour into a greased and floured loaf pan. Bake for about 40 minutes or until toothpick tests done. Serve warm with honey-lemon butter. Yum!

Crusty Tarragon Bread

Tarragon lends a subtle anise flavor to this bread, which is delicious topped with butter, a thin slice of Swiss cheese, and fresh snipped chives!

7½ c. all-purpose flour

5 tsp. active dry yeast

1½ c. milk, divided

2 Tbsp. sugar

2 Tbsp. butter

1 tsp. dried onions

2 tsp. salt

10¾ oz. condensed cream of potato soup

½ c. sour cream

1 Tbsp. snipped fresh or 1 tsp. dried tarragon

Warm ½ cup of milk to about 125°; dissolve yeast in warm milk. In a saucepan, heat and stir remaining milk, sugar, butter, and salt until butter barely melts. Stir in dried onions, soup, sour cream, yeast mixture, and tarragon. Add 3 cups flour and beat well for about 1 minute. Stir in as much remaining flour as possible. Turn onto a floured surface and knead for 5 minutes. Place in a greased bowl (turning once to grease top); cover and let rise in a warm place for about 1 hour. Punch dough down. Lightly grease two 2-quart casserole dishes. Divide dough in half and shape into two balls. Place in casserole dishes and cover. Let rise in a warm place for about a half hour. Preheat oven to 375°. Grease tops and bake for 25-28 minutes, or until hollow sounding when you tap the bottom.

Delicious Dill Bread

2 c. all-purpose flour

2½ tsp. active dry yeast

½ c. water

½ c. cottage cheese

1 Tbsp. sugar

1 Tbsp. dill seeds, heaping

1 Tbsp. butter

1 tsp. salt

1 egg, beaten

Grease a 9" round baking dish. In a mixing bowl, combine flour and yeast. In a saucepan, heat water, cottage cheese, sugar, dill seeds, butter, and salt until butter almost melts. Remove from heat and beat in egg. Add to flour mixture and beat with a wooden spoon for about 1 minute. Add more flour if needed to make a stiff batter. Spoon into prepared pan. Cover and let rise in a warm place for about 1 hour. Preheat oven to 375°. Bake for 25-30 minutes or until golden. Serve warm and spread with butter.

Fennel Seed Quick Bread

And it is quick bread—quick to make and quick to disappear! Serve warm, smothered in butter. Try a slice or two with Chilled Fennel Soup (see page 179) for a light and nutritious lunch.

2 c. flour

¾ c. sugar

2 tsp. baking powder

¼ tsp. salt

1 egg, beaten

1 c. milk

½ c. olive oil

1 Tbsp. fennel seeds

Preheat oven to 350°. Grease an 8"x4"x2" loaf pan. In a bowl, combine dry ingredients (except fennel seeds). In another bowl, mix egg, milk, and oil. Gently stir into flour mixture. Fold in fennel seeds. Spoon into loaf pan and bake for 35-40 minutes, or until a toothpick comes out clean.

Yummy Chive Muffins

These melt-in-your-mouth tender muffins burst with flavor and are the perfect accompaniment to quiches, soups, and chowders.

2⅛ c. all-purpose flour

3 tsp. baking powder

¼ tsp. salt

2 eggs

1 c. milk

2 Tbsp. olive oil

½ c. crumbled feta cheese

¼ c. snipped fresh chives

Preheat oven to 400°. Combine dry ingredients. In a separate bowl, mix eggs, milk, and oil; stir gently into dry ingredients. Fold in feta cheese and chives. Fill greased muffin cups ⅔ full. Bake for 18-20 minutes or until toothpick comes out clean. Serve warm. Refrigerate leftovers.

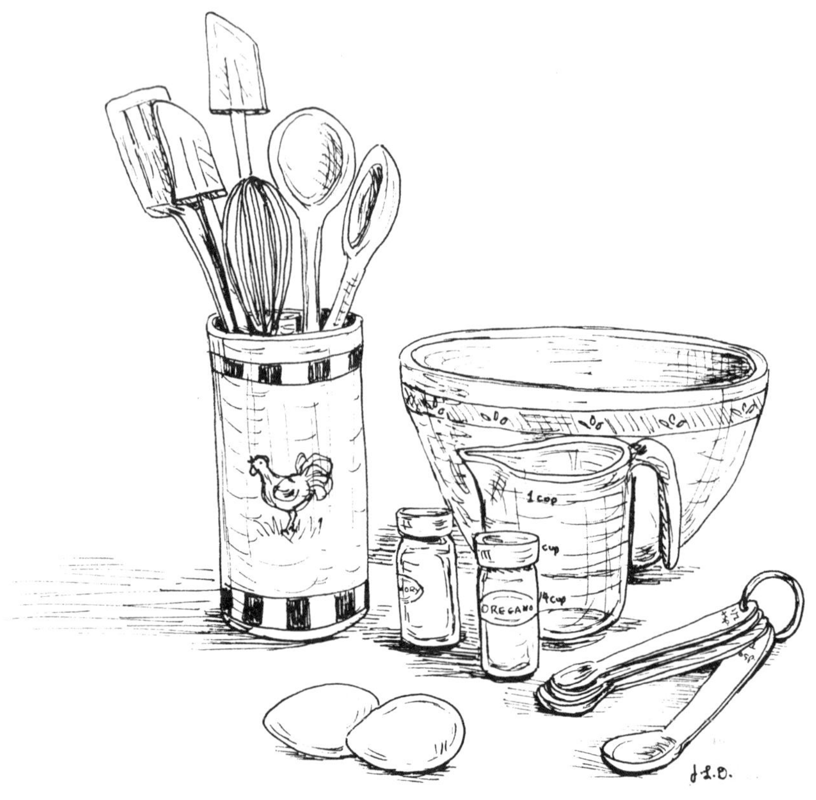

Good-Morning Marjoram Egg Biscuits

3 c. all-purpose flour

1 Tbsp. baking powder

1 tsp. sugar

¼ tsp. salt

¾ tsp. cream of tartar

¾ c. cold butter

1 c. milk

2 Tbsp. chopped fresh marjoram, or 2 tsp. dry

Preheat oven to 450°. In a bowl, combine flour, baking powder, sugar, salt, cream of tartar (and, if using dried, marjoram). Cut in butter until mixture looks like crumbs. Add milk and stir in gently. If using fresh marjoram, fold in. Knead gently 5 times. Lightly roll out on a floured surface to about ¾" thick. Cut with a biscuit cutter and place biscuits on an ungreased baking sheet. Bake for 10-15 minutes.

Toppings:

butter

fried eggs

cheddar cheese slices

fresh baby spinach leaves

Assemble, serve alongside fresh fruit, and enjoy!

Hearty Rosemary Biscuits

2 c. all-purpose flour

2 c. whole wheat flour

4 tsp. sugar

½ tsp. salt

2 Tbsp. baking powder

1 tsp. cream of tartar

1⅓ c. milk

¾ c. olive oil

1 Tbsp. finely chopped fresh rosemary leaves

Preheat oven to 400°. Combine dry ingredients. In a separate bowl, combine remaining ingredients, except for rosemary. Add to dry mixture until moistened; fold in rosemary. Turn on a floured surface and gently knead 5 times. Roll out to ½" thick and cut with a biscuit cutter. Place on ungreased baking sheets and bake for 10-12 minutes. Serve hot with butter alongside soups, stews, roasts, or Italian dishes.

Lavender Honey-Butter

1 Tbsp. ground, dried lavender flowers

8 Tbsp. butter, softened

1 Tbsp. honey

Blend well and spread on warm biscuits or scones.

Cranberry Coriander Scones

Filling:

⅓ c. plus 2 Tbsp. sugar

¼ c. water

1 c. fresh or frozen cranberries

Dough:

3 c. flour

4 Tbsp. sugar

½ tsp. finely ground coriander seed

3¾ tsp. baking powder

¾ tsp. salt

5½ Tbsp. cold butter

⅓ c. plus 2 Tbsp. milk

1 egg, lightly beaten

2 Tbsp. sugar, divided

In a saucepan, place ⅓ cup plus 2 Tbsp. sugar and ¼ cup water; bring to a boil; add cranberries and boil gently for about 10 minutes, stirring occasionally. Cool. Preheat oven to 400°. In a bowl, combine flour, 4 Tbsp. sugar, ground coriander seed, baking powder, and salt. Cut in butter until crumbly. Combine milk and egg; stir lightly into flour mixture. Knead about 10 times. In a greased glass pie dish, spread half the dough; sprinkle with 1 Tbsp. sugar; spread with cranberry mixture. On a lightly floured surface, pat remaining dough into a circle; place on top of cranberry filling and pinch edges to seal. Sprinkle top with 1 Tbsp. sugar. Using a sharp knife, mark pieces (cutting through the top crust only). Bake for about 15-17 minutes or until light brown on the bottom.

Caraway Scones

These are mouth-wateringly good served with butter or cheese alongside scrambled eggs, soups, or stews.

2 c. all-purpose flour

5 tsp. sugar

2 tsp. dried onions

1 tsp. dill weed

2 tsp. caraway seeds

1 tsp. baking powder

½ tsp. salt

½ tsp. baking soda

6 Tbsp. cold butter

1 egg

¾ c. sour cream

½ c. ricotta cheese

Preheat oven to 400°. Mix dry ingredients; cut in butter until crumbly. In a separate bowl, whisk egg, sour cream, and ricotta cheese. Stir into crumb mixture. Knead gently 5 times. On a greased baking sheet, pat dough into 2 flat circles. Cut each into 6 wedges. Bake for 15-20 minutes or until golden.

[He]... giveth food to all flesh: for his mercy endureth for ever (Psalm 136:25).

Herb Main Dishes

Roasted Chicken

3 lb. chicken, thoroughly rinsed inside and out

2 tsp. salt

1 tsp. paprika

1 tsp. garlic salt

1 tsp. dried thyme

1 onion, peeled and chopped

Combine seasonings and rub all over chicken. Fill cavity with chopped onion. Place chicken in roasting pan; add 1 cup water. Cover and bake at 325° for about 2 hours; remove lid and bake for another hour or until juices run clear.

Creamy Baked Chicken

6 boneless, skinless chicken breast halves

¼ c. all-purpose flour

2 Tbsp. plus 1 tsp. olive oil

3 cloves garlic, minced

½ onion, diced

2 c. whipping cream

½ c. grated Parmesan cheese

1 Tbsp. chopped fresh parsley

Preheat oven to 350°. Place flour in a resealable plastic bag. Add chicken and shake to coat. Place 2 Tbsp. olive oil in a large skillet over medium heat until hot. Add chicken; cook for 10 minutes, turning once. Remove and place in a 13"x9" baking dish. In the same skillet, add 1 tsp. olive oil, garlic, and onions; cook over low heat until tender (about 2 minutes). Increase heat to medium, add whipping cream, Parmesan, and parsley. Cook until smooth, about 2 minutes. Pour over chicken in baking dish; cover with foil. Place in oven and bake for about 30 minutes; remove foil and bake for 15 more minutes.

Bay-Seasoned Pot Roast

1 tsp. garlic salt

4 lb. beef roast

¼ c. olive oil

1 large onion, peeled and finely chopped

2 garlic cloves, minced

¼ tsp. dried thyme

2 Tbsp. dried onions

2 dried bay leaves, whole

¼ c. Worcestershire sauce

2 c. water

Preheat oven to 325°. Rub garlic salt into roast; brown in a skillet in oil. Combine diced onion and garlic cloves in a roasting pan. Add roast, turning to coat with mixture. Sprinkle with thyme and dried onions, and lay bay leaves on top (do not crumble). Combine water and Worcestershire sauce; pour over roast. Bake for about 3 hours. Remove bay leaves. Serve and enjoy!

Grilled Herbed Burgers

1 egg, beaten

¼ c. chopped onion

2 Tbsp. dry bread crumbs

2 Tbsp. snipped fresh basil

1 clove garlic, minced

1 lb. ground beef

Combine; shape into four patties. Grill for 20-25 minutes, turning once halfway through grilling. Serve on toasted whole wheat bread spread with butter. Top with lettuce, tomato slices, fresh spinach leaves, and fresh basil leaves.

Dill and Chive Salmon

2 tsp. snipped fresh dill or ¾ tsp. dill weed

½ tsp. lemon-pepper seasoning

¼ tsp. garlic powder

¼ c. packed brown sugar

3 Tbsp. water

3 Tbsp. olive oil

3 Tbsp. soy sauce

3 Tbsp. snipped fresh chives

1 small lemon, thinly sliced

½ onion, sliced

1 salmon fillet, about 1½ pounds

Put all ingredients (except salmon, lemon, and onion slices) in a resealable plastic bag. Combine well. Add salmon and refrigerate for 1 hour, turning once to make sure marinade permeates the salmon. Discard marinade. Place salmon (skin side down) on grill over medium-low heat; top with lemon and onion slices. Cover and cook for 25-30 minutes or until fish flakes with a fork. Another option is to bake the salmon: Discard marinade; place salmon in a greased baking dish; top with lemon and onion slices; cover and bake at 350° for about 20-25 minutes.

Unbeatable Stuffing

Here's a poultry stuffing that adds "Mmmmm, yum!"s and "Ahhh—tasty!"s to the dinner table!

½ lb. Italian sausage
4 c. seasoned stuffing cubes
1½ c. crushed corn bread stuffing
½ c. chopped pecans
½ c. minced fresh parsley
1 Tbsp. minced fresh sage
2½ c. sliced baby portobello mushrooms
1 large onion, peeled and chopped
2 celery ribs, sliced
3 Tbsp. butter, for sautéing
3 Tbsp. butter, to dot stuffing with when cooking
12 oz. chicken broth

In a large skillet, cook sausage until no longer pink; drain well. Place in a bowl; add stuffing cubes, corn bread stuffing, pecans, parsley, and sage. In the skillet, sauté mushrooms, onion, and celery in butter for 5 minutes. Stir into stuffing mixture; add broth. Transfer to a large saucepan. Dot with remaining butter. Cover and cook on low for about 45 minutes, stirring occasionally.

Fennel Sausage Patties

Tasty alongside a stack of buttery pancakes!

2 lb. ground pork

1½ tsp. fennel seed

½ Tbsp. dried parsley, crushed

2 tsp. salt

2 tsp. paprika

1 tsp. garlic powder

¼ tsp. allspice

½ tsp. ground black pepper

1 Tbsp. packed brown sugar

Combine dry ingredients; mix with pork. Form into patties and fry for about 15-20 minutes (or until no longer pink inside).

Baked Garlic

Baking whole garlic heads tones down the flavor but doesn't hinder the powerful healing properties! Blend warm cloves with softened butter and spread onto slices of bread, baked potatoes, or top a steaming mound of mashed potatoes.

1 bulb garlic, unpeeled

2 tsp. olive oil

Place garlic bulb in a small baking dish. Pour olive oil over the garlic. Cover dish with foil. Bake at 350° for about an hour or until soft. Allow garlic to cool, remove foil, and gently squeeze roasted cloves out of peel.

Brown Rice with Mint and Chives

2 c. brown rice, cooked and kept hot

1 c. slivered almonds

2 Tbsp. fresh snipped chives

2 Tbsp. fresh mint, finely chopped

4 Tbsp. olive oil

Stir together and serve hot. Deliciously different!

Chinese "Five-Spice Powder"

This yummy blend goes well with meat, sausage, poultry, and fish.

3 Tbsp. ground cinnamon

6 star anise or 2 Tbsp. anise seeds

1½ tsp. fennel seeds

1½ tsp. whole black peppercorns

¾ tsp. ground cloves

In a blender combine all ingredients. Cover and blend until powdery. Store in an airtight container.

Dill Veggies

1 Tbsp. olive oil

3 c. broccoli florets

2 c. fresh mushrooms of choice

dash of salt

½ tsp. garlic powder

2 tsp. fresh dill, snipped, or ½ tsp. dried dillweed

2 tomatoes, diced

2 Tbsp. lemon juice

¼ c. chicken broth

In a skillet, heat oil over medium heat. Add broccoli, mushrooms, salt, and garlic. Cook and stir for about 10 minutes. Add tomatoes, broth, lemon juice, and dill. Heat thoroughly.

Bread Crumb Mix

This is perfect for breading chicken or fish!

2 slices whole wheat bread, torn

½ c. sliced almonds

2 Tbsp. fresh snipped basil

2 Tbsp. fresh chopped parsley

2 cloves garlic, minced

½ tsp. salt

Place in a blender and blend until coarsely chopped. Coat meat with oil; gently press with bread crumb mixture before baking.

Rosemary Chops

½ c. soy sauce

½ c. water

3 Tbsp. brown sugar

1 tsp. dried rosemary, crushed

4 boneless pork loin chops

In a large resealable plastic bag, combine all ingredients. Seal bag; shake gently to blend. Refrigerate for at least 3 hours, turning to coat. Drain and discard marinade. Place chops in a greased baking dish and bake, uncovered, at 350° for about an hour. Yield: 4 servings.

Herb Salads

Garlicky Cucumber Side

3 cucumbers, peeled, sliced, and cubed
1 clove garlic, peeled and crushed
¼ tsp. ground black pepper
½ tsp. ground ginger
¼ c. diced onion
¼ c. fresh snipped chives
1 c. plain yogurt

Combine; refrigerate for at least an hour. Serve cold alongside hamburgers and steak fries.

Garden-Fresh Potato Salad

3 lb. fingerling potatoes, washed and cut into thirds
2 Tbsp. olive oil
½ tsp. coarse ground sea salt
1 large sweet red pepper, chopped
1 medium red onion, peeled and diced
1 medium cucumber, chopped
2 small zucchini, chopped
1 c. cherry tomatoes, halved
¾ c. vinaigrette
½ c. halved Greek olives
2¼ oz. sliced ripe olives, drained
2 Tbsp. fresh oregano, or 2 tsp. dried

In an electric skillet, add olive oil, potatoes, and salt; toss to coat. Cook at 350°, stirring occasionally, for about 20 minutes. Place in a large bowl. Add other ingredients and toss to coat. Place in refrigerator until cold. Delicious!

Sage Fritters

oil for deep-frying

25 fresh sage leaves

1 c. all-purpose flour

2 Tbsp. olive oil

4 Tbsp. water

1 egg white

Rinse (and gently pat dry) sage leaves; set aside. Mix all other ingredients except oil for frying. Place oil for frying in a large skillet. When hot, dip leaves in batter one at a time. Fry several at a time for 1-2 minutes each (until golden). Drain briefly on paper towels. Place in a baking dish and keep warm in oven until done frying all leaves. Serve warm with salt and pepper. Side dish for 5.

Best Macaroni Salad

2 c. cooked elbow macaroni

15 oz. garbanzo beans, rinsed and drained

4 hard-boiled eggs, chopped

½ c. chopped dill pickles

½ c. mayonnaise

⅛ c. chopped onion

3 Tbsp. fresh minced parsley

½ c. sliced ripe olives

1 Tbsp. mustard seed

2 Tbsp. pickle juice

¼ tsp. garlic powder

salt and pepper to taste

Combine all ingredients, tossing to coat. Cover and refrigerate for at least an hour. Yield: 8 servings.

Savory White Bean Salad

1 onion, peeled and chopped

3 cloves garlic, peeled and minced

1 Tbsp. olive oil

1 Tbsp. chopped fresh savory

19 oz. white kidney or navy beans, rinsed and drained

14½ oz. diced tomatoes, drained, reserving ½ c.

2 slices bacon, cooked, drained, and crumbled

salad greens

vinaigrette

In a skillet, sauté onion and garlic in olive oil for about 3 minutes. Stir in beans and savory. Mix in tomatoes and reserved juice. Cook and stir over medium heat until thoroughly heated. Remove from heat and mix in bacon bits. Arrange salad greens on 4 plates; top with bean mixture. Drizzle with vinaigrette.

Refreshingly Minty Fruit Salad

1 c. halved red or purple grapes

2 apples, cored and diced

1 banana, sliced

2 ripe peaches, peeled and sliced

1 ripe pear, peeled and sliced

1 c. hulled and sliced fresh strawberries

1 c. small marshmallows

3 Tbsp. strong mint tea with 1 tsp. honey

2 c. whipped topping

Combine fruit. Stir in honey-sweetened mint tea. Let stand for 20 minutes. Stir in whipped topping; fold in marshmallows. Place in 6 bowls. Garnish each serving with fresh mint leaves. Serve immediately.

Soups & Sandwiches

Cilantro Soup

4 c. chicken broth

16 oz. frozen vegetables

15 oz. black beans, rinsed and drained

15 oz. pinto beans, rinsed and drained

14½ oz. diced tomatoes, undrained

1 sweet onion, chopped

1½ Tbsp. chili powder

1 Tbsp. minced fresh cilantro

4 cloves garlic, minced

½ c. fresh chopped chives, reserve for sprinkling over soup

½ c. grated cheddar cheese, reserve for sprinkling over soup

1 c. sour cream

In a kettle, combine all ingredients except chives, cheese, and sour cream. Bring to a boil over medium heat; reduce heat to low and simmer for about an hour. Serve sprinkled with chives and cheese; top with a spoonful of sour cream. Yield: 6 servings.

Healthy-Thyme Soup

7 medium carrots, grated

3 pt. chicken stock

1 lb. cooked leftover chicken breast, chopped

1 sweet onion, chopped

1 clove garlic, minced

2 tsp. dried thyme, or 4 tsp. fresh

Bring to a boil. Simmer in a covered saucepan for about half an hour. Delicious on a cold winter day! Yield: 6 servings.

Creamy Salmon Thyme Chowder

1 c. frozen broccoli
1 c. frozen corn
1 Tbsp. butter
½ onion, peeled and chopped
2 Tbsp. all-purpose flour
2 c. milk
1 c. light cream
2 c. frozen loose-pack hash brown potatoes
15 oz. salmon fillet, cooked and flaked, or
  15 oz. canned salmon, drained and flaked
¼ c. fresh snipped parsley
1 Tbsp. finely chopped fresh thyme
2 Tbsp. lemon juice

In a kettle, cook frozen vegetables and onion in butter; stir in flour. Stir in milk and cream. Cook and stir until bubbly. Remove from heat. Stir in thawed hash brown potatoes, salmon, parsley, thyme, and lemon juice. Cook and stir until heated through. Serve with oyster crackers and a big salad, sprinkled with fresh lemon thyme leaves, of course!

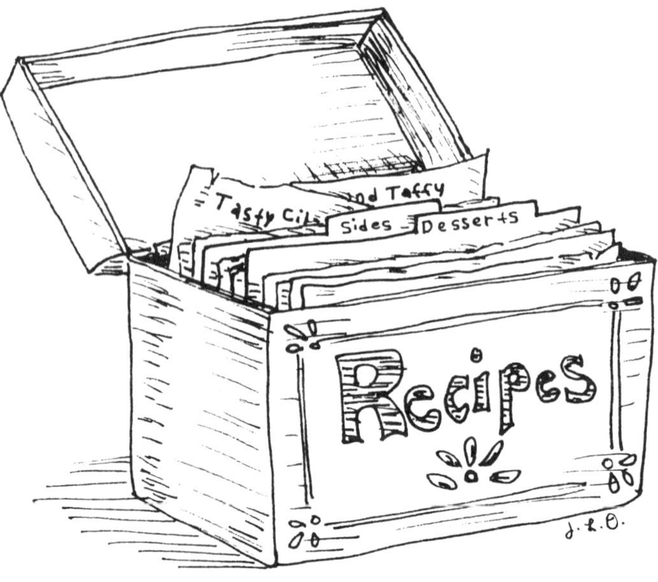

After-Thanksgiving Turkey Soup

Need to use up leftover turkey? Here's the perfect solution!

1 onion, peeled and chopped

3 celery ribs with leaves, cut in small pieces

8 Tbsp. butter

7 Tbsp. all-purpose flour

¼ tsp. garlic powder

1 Tbsp. fresh chopped parsley

½ tsp. dried thyme

1½ c. milk

4 c. chopped turkey

6 carrots, washed and sliced

1½-2 c. turkey broth

2 c. frozen corn, thawed

In a kettle, sauté onion and celery in butter for about 5 minutes. Stir in flour and seasonings; gradually add milk, stirring constantly until smooth and thickened. Add turkey and carrots. Add broth (as much as needed for desired consistency). Bring to a boil, stirring constantly; immediately lower heat, cover, and simmer for 30 minutes. Add thawed corn and simmer for 15 minutes more. Makes about 8 servings.

Chilled Fennel Soup

2½ c. plain yogurt

3 Tbsp. ice water

1 Tbsp. chopped fennel leaves

3 tomatoes, peeled and thinly sliced

3 hard-boiled eggs, sliced

Combine all ingredients except hard-boiled eggs. Ladle into 3 bowls and top with sliced eggs. Salt and pepper to taste.

Bay Beef Broth

This broth is good added to soups, stews, and in dishes that call for beef broth. The flavor of bay is predominant, which gives it its name.

4 lb. meaty beef soup bones
2 Tbsp. olive oil
¾ c. water
3 large carrots, sliced
1 large onion, peeled and diced
2 celery stalks with leaves, sliced
½ Tbsp. dried basil, crushed
10 whole black peppercorns
10 sprigs fresh parsley
5 dried bay leaves, whole
2 cloves garlic, peeled and halved
10 c. water

In a roasting pan, place oil and the soup bones. Bake at 450° for about 30 minutes, turning once. Place bones in a kettle. Pour ¾ cup water in the roasting pan, and scrape up browned bits; pour (while scraping carefully) into the kettle. Stir in remaining ingredients. Bring to a boil, then simmer, covered, for 3-4 hours. Remove soup bones. Strain broth through a large colander layered with cheesecloth. Chill; skim off fat. Use immediately, or place broth in a sealed container and refrigerate for up to 3 days, or freeze for up to 6 months. Makes about 8 cups.

Fennel Crackers

¼ tsp. fennel seed, crushed

3 black peppercorns, crushed

1 c. whole wheat flour

1 tsp. baking powder

1 tsp. soy sauce

¼ c. lemon juice

enough water to form a dough

Preheat oven to 350°. Mix together dry ingredients; mix liquids and pour over dry. Gently stir with a fork, sprinkling in water as needed until a ball can be formed. Divide in half; roll out each half on a lightly floured surface to about 1⁄16 inch thick. Cut into squares. Bake squares on a cookie sheet for 8-10 minutes.

Breakfast Egg and Basil Sandwich

1 English muffin, split, toasted, and buttered

1 egg, fried or scrambled

1 slice cheddar cheese

1 slice tomato

8 fresh basil leaves

6 fresh baby spinach leaves

fried ham, sausage, or bacon, optional

Toast and butter muffin. Place cheese on bottom half; add egg and ham, sausage, or bacon; add top half. Wrap in foil and bake until hot and melty. Add tomato, basil, and spinach, with a bit of prepared mustard. Delicious!

Hot and Tangy Fish Sandwiches

6 slices whole wheat bread

3 squares frozen fish fillets, baked according to package directions

3 Tbsp. grated horseradish

1 Tbsp. fresh minced chives

½ c. softened cream cheese

1 Tbsp. sour cream

pinch salt

¼ tsp. cayenne pepper

½ tsp. prepared mustard

tomato slices, spinach leaves, alfalfa sprouts

While fish fillets are cooking, combine all ingredients except bread, tomatoes, spinach, and alfalfa sprouts. Toast bread slices and spread with the mixture. Top with fish, tomatoes, spinach, and alfalfa sprouts.

Sage Patties

1 lb. ground turkey

¾ tsp. salt

½ tsp. dried, crushed sage

½ tsp. dried thyme

¼ tsp. ground nutmeg, if desired

¼ tsp. cayenne pepper

olive oil

Mix together all ingredients except oil. Shape into patties. Pour about 2 tsp. oil in a large skillet; cook patties in hot oil over medium heat for 15 minutes, turning once. Yield: about 8 patties.

Herb Dips, Sauces, & Spreads

Tasty Cilantro Dip

So-o-o good served with tortilla and corn chips! Delicious for topping tacos, tostadas, and burritos. Try it on rice too!

½ c. diced onion

2 tomatoes, chopped

2 oz. diced green chilies

¼ c. tomato paste

¼ c. lime juice

¼ tsp. salt

½ c. fresh cilantro, finely chopped

Combine all ingredients. Cover and refrigerate for at least 3 hours to blend flavors.

Creamy Tarragon Veggie Dip

6 oz. softened cream cheese

2 Tbsp. milk, or more

2 Tbsp. fresh tarragon, finely chopped, or 2 tsp. dried tarragon

1 clove garlic, peeled and chopped

Blend well. Refrigerate overnight in a sealed container. Serve as a dip for veggies, spread for crackers, or tasty topping for fresh-baked whole wheat bread!

Dilly Dip

This tasty dip incorporates fresh dill leaves into a creamy mixture that's perfect for fresh vegetables,crackers, and corn chips!

8 oz. cream cheese, softened
8 oz. sour cream
2 Tbsp. snipped fresh chives
2 Tbsp. snipped fresh dill,
  or 2 tsp. dried dill weed
¼ tsp. salt

Combine ingredients; beat with spoon until fluffy. Cover and chill for an hour. Add 1-2 Tbsp. of milk for desired consistency. Serve cold and refrigerate leftovers.

Herb Cheese Spread

1 Tbsp. each of chopped, fresh
chives
thyme
oregano
basil
parsley
8 oz. cream cheese, softened

Blend well; refrigerate overnight. Spread over crackers, on sandwiches, and, if you whip in 3 Tbsp. sour cream, use as a vegetable dip.

The "Real" Pizza Sauce!

Oregano is that "secret" ingredient which gives pizza sauce its "pizza" flavor. Here's the recipe we like best.

14½ oz. diced tomatoes

6 oz. tomato paste

1 tsp. olive oil

1 tsp. sugar

½ tsp. dried basil

½ tsp. salt

1 tsp. garlic powder

1 tsp. dried oregano

¼ tsp. dried thyme

Combine sauce ingredients in a bowl. Spread over two 14" pizza crusts. Add favorite toppings and bake according to pizza recipe.

Tomato Basil Sauce

1 c. chopped onion

2 cloves garlic, minced

2 Tbsp. butter

28 oz. canned tomatoes, cut up

⅓ c. tomato paste

¼ tsp. sugar

½ c. fresh basil

In a saucepan combine onion, garlic, and butter. Cook until tender. Stir in tomatoes, tomato paste, and sugar. Bring mixture to a boil over medium-low heat. Simmer on low, uncovered, for about 15 minutes. Stir in basil. Simmer 5 more minutes. Makes about 3 cups of super-delicious sauce that perks up pasta dishes, and makes a nice beef soup base and a tasty meat loaf sauce!

Coriander Seed Pickling Spice

2½ tsp. dried coriander seed

5 dried bay leaves

2¼ tsp. dill seed

2 Tbsp. mustard seed

2 tsp. black peppercorns

2¼ tsp. allspice

Combine in an airtight container or resealable bag. Makes about ⅓ cup (good for 2 gallons).

When making refrigerator pickles, you will need:

2 Tbsp. sugar

1 onion, peeled and chopped

2 bunches fresh dill

2 cloves garlic, peeled and halved

6 dozen small cucumbers

⅔ c. canning salt

1 qt. vinegar

1 qt. water

Loosely pack pickles in a sterilized, hot wide-mouth 2-gallon glass canning jar. Add onion, garlic cloves, and Coriander Seed Pickling Spice mix. Layer with fresh dill. In a saucepan, combine vinegar, water, salt, and sugar; bring to a boil; pour over pickles. Seal with a lid. Allow to cool completely, then refrigerate for 2 weeks before opening. Keep refrigerated after opening, and use within a month.

Classic Pesto

½ c. olive oil

2 c. fresh basil leaves, packed

½ c. pine nuts

¾ c. grated Parmesan cheese

4 cloves garlic, peeled and quartered

Place in a blender; cover and blend (scraping the sides) until almost smooth. Place in saucepan and warm over low heat, if desired. Use immediately. Traditionally poured over cooked and drained pasta, and tossed to coat. Also good served with fish, over fresh-picked, steamed green beans, or used in pasta soups. Makes about 1 cup pesto. For variety, add ½ cup parsley (packed) and 2 Tbsp. melted butter to the above recipe. This makes a yummy sandwich spread!

Best-Ever Guacamole

4 ripe avocados, peeled, seeded, and mashed

2 tomatoes, chopped

½ c. diced onion

¼ c. fresh cilantro, finely chopped

½ tsp. dried oregano

⅛ tsp. garlic powder

Combine all ingredients. Cover and refrigerate for about 1 hour. Serve with tortilla chips or Mexican entrées. Also tasty as a spread for chicken sandwiches and hamburgers.

Bright Orange Horseradish Sauce

The combination of ketchup and mustard give this sauce its vibrant color.

¾ c. ketchup

2 Tbsp. fresh grated horseradish root

1 Tbsp. prepared mustard

Combine and serve with hot dogs, burgers, fish, or steak fries.

Horseradish Sauce

This sauce is a tasty variation from typical spreads like mayonnaise. It's also a good dipping sauce for fish!

1 c. cold whipping cream

4 Tbsp. freshly grated horseradish root

3 tsp. lemon juice

½ onion, peeled and finely chopped

Beat cream with an electric mixer until thick. Gently fold in the other ingredients. Refrigerate for an hour; gently whisk before serving.

Mint Pancake Syrup

This is especially good drizzled generously over strawberry and whipped cream topped pancakes.

¾ c. fresh mint leaves

1 c. water

2 c. sugar

Tear up mint leaves and place in a saucepan with water and sugar. Mix well. Bring to a boil, stirring constantly. Reduce heat to low and simmer, stirring occasionally, for about 10 minutes. Strain out leaves and serve warm. Cool leftovers and store in the refrigerator. If desired, you may add the cooled syrup to lemonade and iced tea, or use as sweetener for hot tea.

Easy Mint Jelly Sauce

Good served hot over pork, or used to top toasted English muffins or bread.

1 Tbsp. chopped mint

1 c. jelly of your choice (strawberry is good!)

Place in a saucepan and stir over very low heat until heated through. Let cool slightly and use immediately.

Salmon Parsley Spread

8 oz. cream cheese spread

2 Tbsp. minced onion

1 Tbsp. lemon juice

1 tsp. prepared horseradish

½ tsp. prepared mustard

14½ oz. canned salmon, drained, bones and skin removed

2 Tbsp. fresh minced parsley

Blend first 5 ingredients; fold in salmon. Sprinkle with parsley. This is perfect as a sandwich spread or cracker topping.

Salad Dressing

2 c. sour cream

1 tsp. fresh, chopped parsley

1 tsp. fresh, chopped chives

1 tsp. fresh, chopped tarragon

2 Tbsp. brown sugar

¼ c. apple cider vinegar

¼ c. olive oil

1 tsp. dry mustard

In a large jar with a tightly fitting lid, combine all ingredients. Lasts (refrigerated) for up to a week; shake well before using.

Desserts with Herbs

Coriander Sugar Cookies

Crisp, flaky, and delightful served with a cup of hot tea, or alongside a tall glass of lemonade.

1 c. granulated sugar
¼ tsp. salt
¾ c. butter, softened
1 egg
1 tsp. vanilla extract
1 tsp. grated lemon rind
3 c. all-purpose flour
1 tsp. baking powder
¼ tsp. finely ground coriander seed
granulated sugar to sprinkle on cookies

Preheat oven to 350°. Cream together sugar, salt, and butter. Beat egg, lemon rind, and extract into creamed mixture until fluffy. In a separate bowl, mix flour, baking powder, and ground coriander seed. Stir into creamed mixture. Roll ⅛" thick on a floured board. Cut into circles with biscuit cutter (or use shaped cookie cutters, if desired). Arrange on an ungreased baking sheet. Sprinkle with sugar. Bake for 9-10 minutes or until golden at the edges. Remove and cool completely. About 4 dozen cookies.

Caraway Biscotti

Not too sweet, deliciously crisp, and wonderful served with a steaming cup of hot tea!

3⅔ c. all-purpose flour

4 tsp. baking soda

pinch salt

2 tsp. bruised caraway seeds

½ tsp. cinnamon

¼ tsp. ground nutmeg

2 eggs

2 Tbsp. milk

⅓ c. honey

½ c. melted butter

Preheat oven to 325°. Mix dry ingredients. In a separate bowl, beat eggs and milk; whisk in honey and butter. Add to dry ingredients (add more milk if needed). Knead gently 5 times. Shape into two 10" long logs. Place on a greased baking sheet and bake for 18 minutes or until golden. Remove from oven and reduce heat to 275°. When loaves are cool, slice into ½" slices and arrange flat on greased baking sheets. Bake for 8 minutes; turn and bake for 5-8 minutes longer or until golden. Cool completely. If desired, dip one end in melted chocolate chips. Let dry completely. Store in an airtight container for up to 3 weeks in the refrigerator.

Lavender Sprinkles

1 c. ground, dried lavender blossoms

1 c. granulated sugar

Combine and mix well. Roll sugar cookies in this mixture before baking. Sprinkle mixture over white-frosted cupcakes. Scatter over buttered pancakes.

Lemon Balm Cheesecake Dessert

Pastry:

1 c. flour

⅛ tsp. salt

4 Tbsp. cold butter, cut into pieces

Filling:

4 Tbsp. butter, softened

2 Tbsp. honey

12 oz. cream cheese, softened

2 eggs, beaten

6 Tbsp. finely chopped lemon balm

Preheat oven to 400°. For pastry, cut butter into flour and salt mixture; add enough water to make a soft dough. (Handle as gently as possible!) Roll out and line a 7-inch quiche dish. Bake for about 10-15 minutes, or until golden brown. Let cool completely. Reduce oven temperature to 350°. Beat butter, honey, and cream cheese; beat in eggs; fold in lemon balm. Pour filling into pastry shell. Bake for 45 minutes or until filling is golden. Yield: 6 servings.

Lemon Balm Lemonade Treats

Lemon balm is soothing to the nerves and stress-related digestive troubles. It relieves sore throats and suppresses coughs. These tasty popsicles are a nice treat on a hot summer evening after a busy day—or why not reach for one the next time you feel the sniffles coming on! They're also soothing and healing to suck on if you suffer from a frequent dry cough.

2 c. water

1 c. packed brown sugar

¼ c. minced fresh lemon balm

¾ c. lemon juice

In a saucepan, mix water and brown sugar; bring to a boil (stirring constantly) and keep on stirring until sugar is dissolved. Remove from heat and stir in lemon balm; cover and steep for 15 minutes. Strain out plant material (if desired). Add lemon juice, stirring well. Cool and pour into paper cups. Freeze slightly; insert sticks. Freeze.

Rosemary Apples

½ tsp. dried rosemary

3 apples, peeled, cored and diced

¼ c. water (more if needed)

¼ c. chopped walnuts

3 Tbsp. packed brown sugar

3 Tbsp. granulated sugar

Combine in a saucepan and simmer until apples are tender. Serve over vanilla ice cream!

Lime Basil Cake

Cake:

1 c. butter, softened

2 c. sugar

2 eggs

½ tsp. vanilla extract

½ tsp. grated lemon peel

3½ c. all-purpose flour

2 tsp. baking powder

1 tsp. baking soda

2 c. sour cream

Lemon-Lime Syrup/Frosting:

1 c. water

¾ c. sugar

⅓ c. lemon juice

10 fresh lime basil leaves

1 large strip lemon peel

Frosting:

1¾ c. confectioners' sugar

3 Tbsp. softened butter

1¼ c. heavy whipping cream

Garnish:

1 tsp. lemon-lime syrup

⅛ c. sugar

new, fine-tipped artist's paintbrush

10 fresh lime basil leaves

Preheat oven to 350°. Cream together butter and sugar; add eggs, beating well after each. Beat in vanilla and lemon peel. In another bowl, mix flour, baking powder, and baking soda. Alternately add flour mixture and sour cream to butter mixture. Pour into two greased and floured 9" round cake pans. Bake for 20-25 minutes (until toothpick comes out clean). Cool 10 minutes. Invert from pans to wire rack; cool completely. The frosting is kind of difficult, but worth it! First make the lemon-lime syrup by combining water, sugar, lemon juice, lime basil, and lemon peel in a saucepan. Bring to a boil; cook over medium-low heat until there is only about 1 cup left. (You'll only need about 4 Tbsp. for this recipe, but save the rest! It's good over pancakes or waffles!) Strain out basil leaves and lemon peel. Cool completely. Meanwhile, whip the cream; set aside. In a mixing bowl, beat the confectioners' sugar, butter, and 3 Tbsp. of lemon-lime syrup. Fold in whipped cream. Lick the spoon—yum! Place one round cake on a serving plate. Frost top; place remaining cake over frosting; frost top and sides. Place in the refrigerator. Now for the garnish! Place 1 Tbsp. lemon-lime syrup in a small bowl. Use the paintbrush to brush the syrup over a basil leaf. Coat with sugar and lay on waxed paper. Repeat with all the leaves. Use to garnish your cake. Serve with your favorite hot beverage and enjoy!

Old-Fashioned Horehound Taffy

1 c. molasses

1 c. granulated sugar

1 c. thin cream

2 Tbsp. butter

1 tsp. baking soda

¾ tsp. horehound concentrate (see following recipe)

Combine molasses, sugar, and cream in a saucepan; bring to a boil over medium heat, stirring constantly. Cook and stir until firm ball stage (244°). Remove from heat and add butter, soda, and horehound concentrate. Stir well. Pour into a greased dish and let cool. You don't have to pull this taffy—simply cut into squares or roll into balls. Delicious!

Horehound Concentrate

This can be used to flavor candies, added to hot water and sweetened with honey as a medicinal drink, or used wherever horehound is added. Horehound's medicinal properties are not diminished when boiling.

2½ tsp. dried horehound

1 c. water

Combine in a small saucepan. Over medium-low heat, bring to a boil. Remove from heat. Cover and steep for 30 minutes. Strain out horehound, squeezing to obtain fullest amount of extract. Return horehound water to low heat and simmer down to concentrate. (Do not allow to scorch!) Cool completely and store in a covered glass jar in the refrigerator for up to two weeks.

Handy Tips for Using Herbs in Your Kitchen

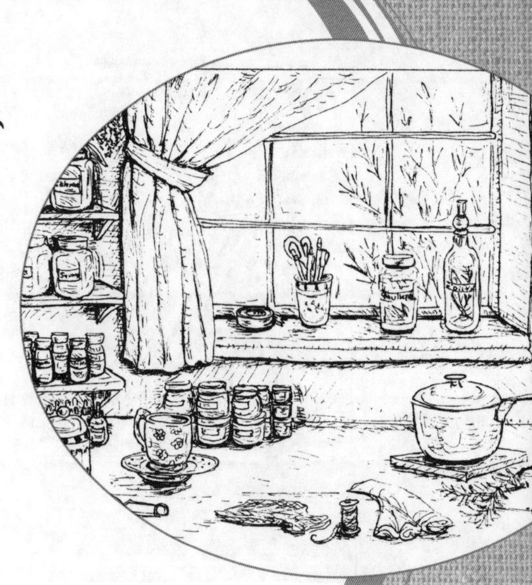

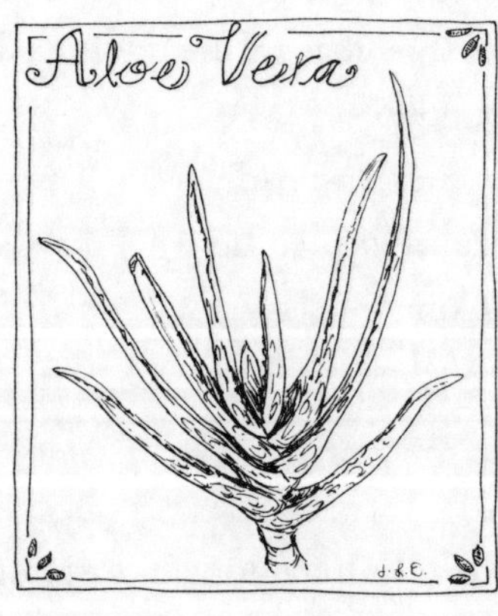

Aloe vera gel is a good base for many essential oils, especially tea tree, lavender, and chamomile.

This herb's highest potency is found in the fresh leaf, used immediately after it is picked. Bottled products make a good "next-best" choice, but only if they are processed in a way that retains the aloe-polysaccharides, with no harmful preservatives added. Read the label before you buy!

· To add a nutritious and healing boost to your shampoos, skin care products, etc., blend in aloe vera gel. A good ratio is 2 tsp. gel for ¼ cup shampoo or cream.

· Smooth on pure aloe vera gel for a quick skin refresher and rejuvenator!

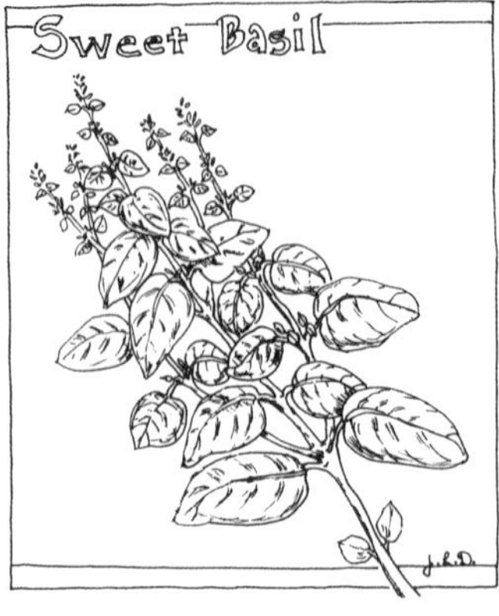

Fresh basil leaves make a flavorful and healthful addition to any tossed green salad. Not only will you love the taste, but you'll be glad to know that the pretty green addition is encouraging healthful digestion!

· Fresh basil lends itself well as a topping for crackers and cream cheese, added to rice, or mixed into fillings for wraps and sandwiches.

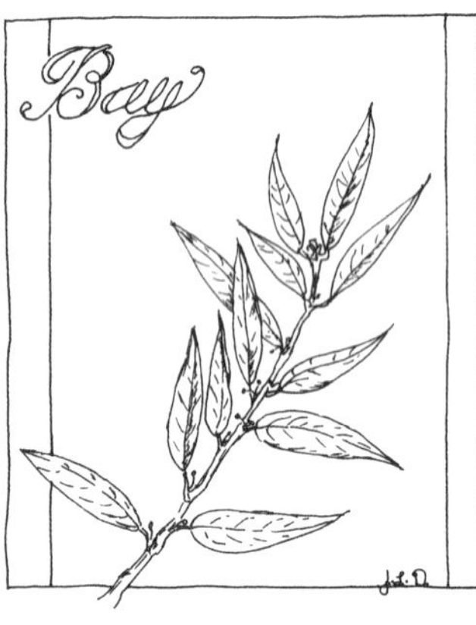

Add a bay leaf to a resealable bag with your favorite marinade. Delicious!

· Bay leaves are sometimes called laurel leaves.

· Bay is the primary ingredient in the traditional *bouquet garni* herb bundle.

· Bay goes deliciously well with garlic!

· BBQ sauce is pleasantly perked up when bay is added during the cooking process.

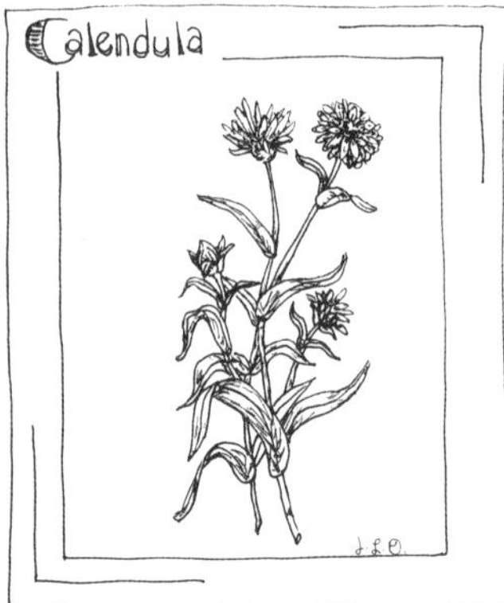

Have a sore, dry scalp? Add half a tsp. of calendula oil to your shampoo. Or infuse dry petals in water and strain; dilute infusion and use as a hair rinse after washing.

· Calendula oil, or a cooled infusion of the petals in water, effectively soothes chicken pox, sunburn, minor skin irritations, rashes, inflammation, and so much more! The tea is a good mouthwash for thrush.

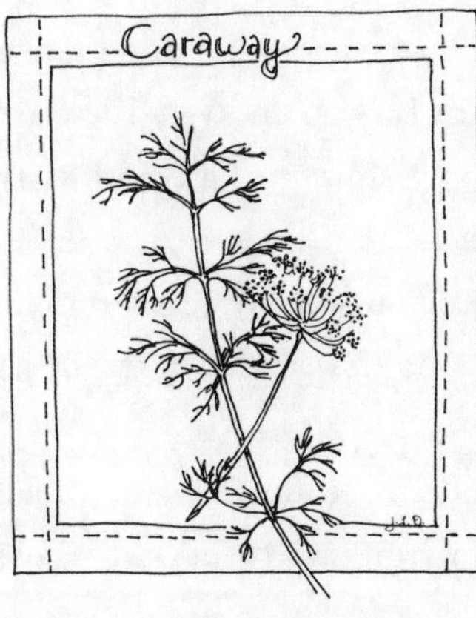

Caraway seeds add a hearty savor to potato-based soups.

· Blend seeds into cream cheese and cheese dips.

· Sprinkle seeds over carrots, beets, turnips, parsnips, or cauliflower before steaming.

· Sauté seeds with onions and mushrooms in butter—delicious!

· Excellent when seeds are sparingly added to apple or raisin desserts. Good with pears and peaches too!

· Mix ½ tsp. seeds into your favorite biscuit recipe.

· Add fresh, young leaves to soups.

· Toss young leaves in green salads!

· Boil or steam roots as you would parsnips.

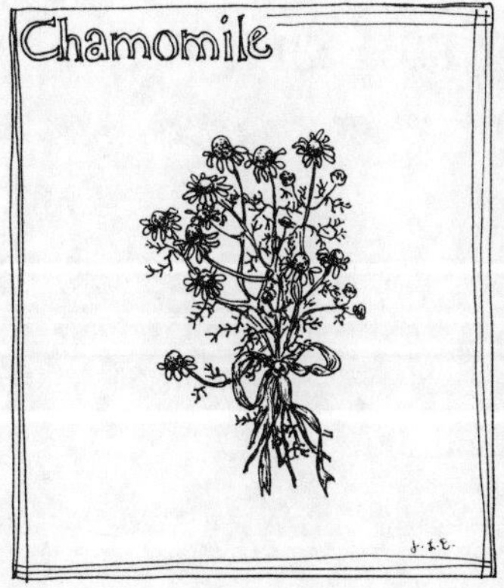

Chamomile tea is so-o-o relaxing! Brew a cup before bed to promote restful sleep.

· Diluted chamomile tea makes a nice hair rinse. It not only adds luster, but helps prevent dandruff and soothe itchy scalps. For added conditioning benefits, include some dried parsley before steeping.

· Remember, chamomile tea bags, slightly cooled, make wonderfully soothing eye compresses that reduce inflammation.

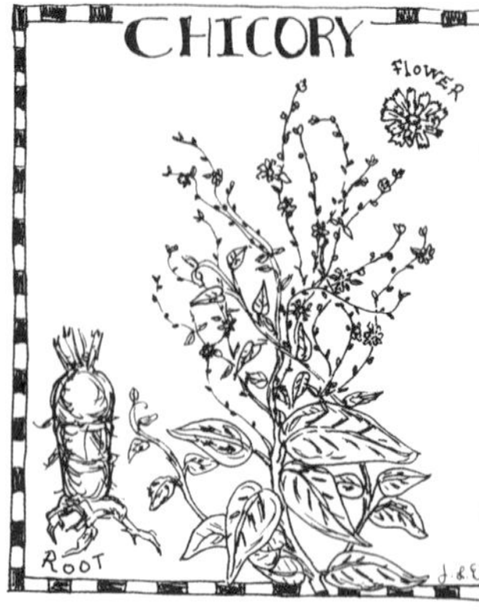

Blanched leaves of chicory are also known as "chicons" or Belgian endive." These are worth the effort to grow, since they are both tasty and nutritious!

· Tender leaves of chicory are used in teas as a tonic for liver troubles. A poultice of the leaves treats inflammation.

· The beautiful lavender-blue flowers are edible. Sprinkle the petals in fruit salads, or add whole flowers as lovely garnishes for cakes and desserts.

· Don't forget that dried chicory root makes a delicious coffee substitute, as well as being a mild laxative and diuretic.

TEN TIPS FOR TOPPING WITH CHIVES

Chives are the ultimate for topping a variety of foods! Here are some of our favorite choices:

· Spoon over Spanish rice before serving.
· Load on tacos.
· Fold into sour cream dips.
· Sprinkle over a baked potato smothered in butter and sour cream.
· Toss in a dinner salad.
· Top potato cheese soup or Mexican soups.
· Scatter thickly over garlic bread before toasting.
· Smother mashed potatoes with freshly snipped chives!
· Top omelets or scrambled eggs.
· Add over fresh salsa for an extra surge of flavor.

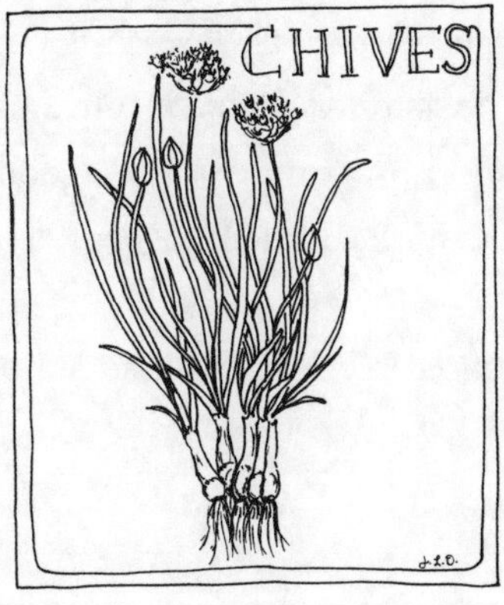

Remember, chive bulbs and flowers are delicious too! Use them fresh, or sauté in butter with mushrooms and serve over hamburgers!

· Chives are best fresh, good dried, but lose most of their flavor when cooked. Add during the last minute or so of cooking, and not before!

· Store fresh chives in the refrigerator in a sealed container for up to 3 days.

· Blend fresh or dried snipped chives into softened cream cheese for a delicious spread.

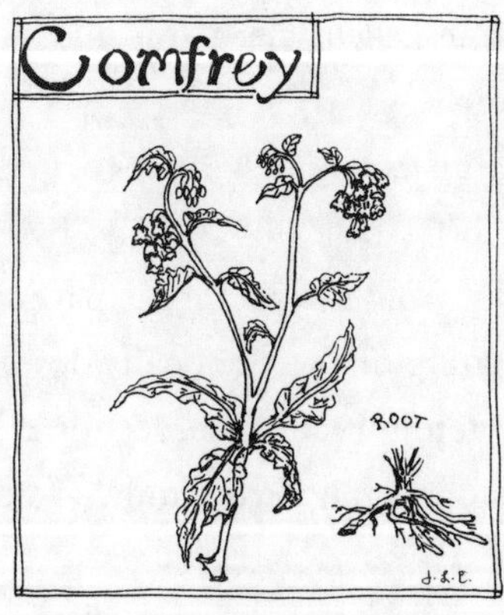

When your comfrey plants begin to die at the end of the season, harvest the leaves and turn into the soil of your potato bed.

· Comfrey is one of the best herbs for infusing in olive oil. The resulting oil is good for treating a number of ailments, including hemorrhoids. You may also use this oil as a rub to heal strained muscles and bruised skin, and it makes an excellent base for ointments.

· Many professionals caution that comfrey should not be taken internally.

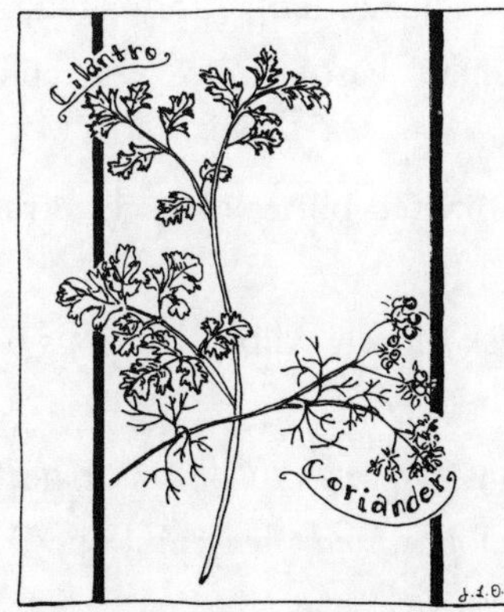

Add ½ Tbsp. of finely ground dried coriander seed to your favorite sweet bread recipe. Serve warm with a honey-butter spread. You'll love it!

· Fresh chopped cilantro is extra good added to green salads and topped with Ranch dressing.

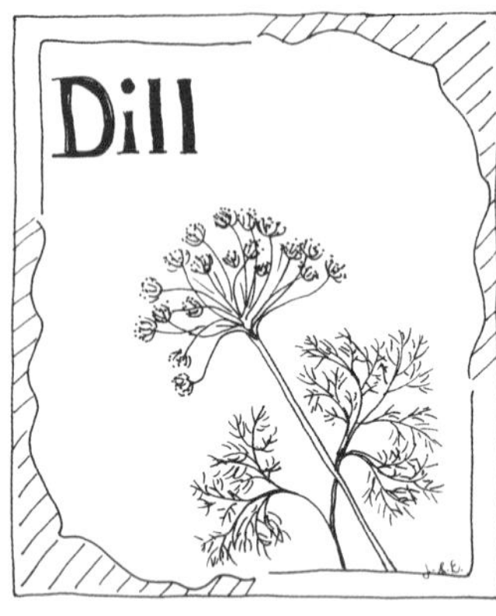

If you like dill pickles, you'll love this! Dip pickle rounds in batter and fry in olive oil until golden brown. Crispy, crunchy, salty—good!

· Fresh dill makes a nice addition to vegetable salads.

· Dill seed and dill weed are wonderful added to potato salads!

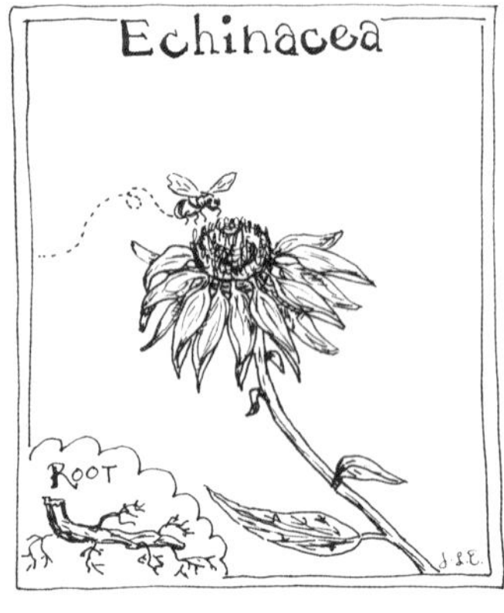

Echinacea is an excellent herb for making healthful tinctures.

· Remember that echinacea is best used to *treat* problems—not to be taken on a daily basis exceeding two-weeks. You may want to have a two-week "off" pattern to one week of daily doses.

· If you suffer from autoimmune disorders or are allergic to members of the ragweed family, avoid echinacea.

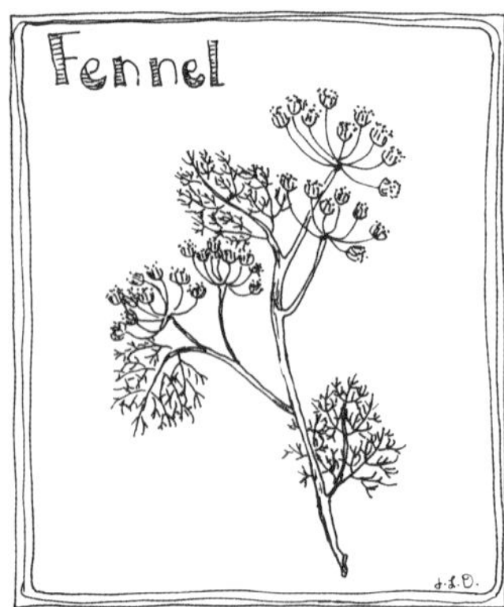

Don't forget the fun idea of using the young, bright green stalks of fennel for drinking straws, tasty with tomato-based chilled vegetable smoothies!

· Blend leaves into softened butter for a flavorful sandwich spread.

· Use the flowerheads as lovely edible additions to fruit or dinner salads!

· Add several teaspoons of dried fennel seeds to beef vegetable soup. Delicious—*and* a healthful boost!

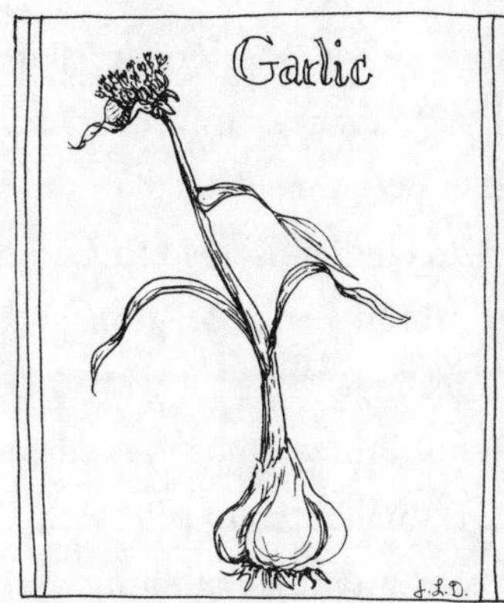

Mash a garlic clove, blend into softened butter, and spread over fish before grilling.

· Before roasting, put small cuts on the top of a beef roast and insert thin slices of garlic cloves.

· Serve sprigs of parsley with garlic dishes—it will sweeten the breath.

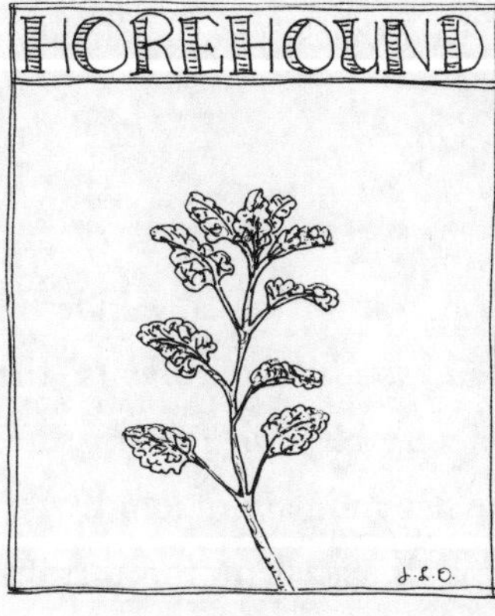

Infuse horehound leaves in milk and pour into saucers. Place on the edges of your deck rails—the mixture attracts and kills flies.

· You can combine crushed aniseed and simmer with horehound leaves in water. Steep, strain, and blend liquid with honey for an effective sore throat remedy.

· Be careful not to consume too much horehound at a time, as it can cause rapid heartbeat. Also, avoid using if pregnant.

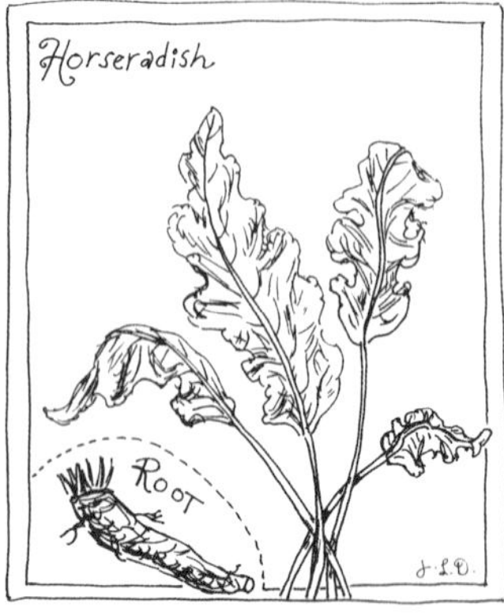

Remember, horseradish can treat skin troubles such as eczema. Infuse grated roots in milk and splash over the affected area for relief. Try the infusion on chilblains, cold feet, and painful joints too. It stimulates circulation and gives a soothing warm feeling.

· Horseradish is powerful! Protect your eyes when grating the root, test on small areas of skin before topical use, and only consume small amounts at a time to prevent heartburn and excessive sweating.

· Add freshly grated horseradish to salad greens for a unique flavor. This snack can help relieve congestion too!

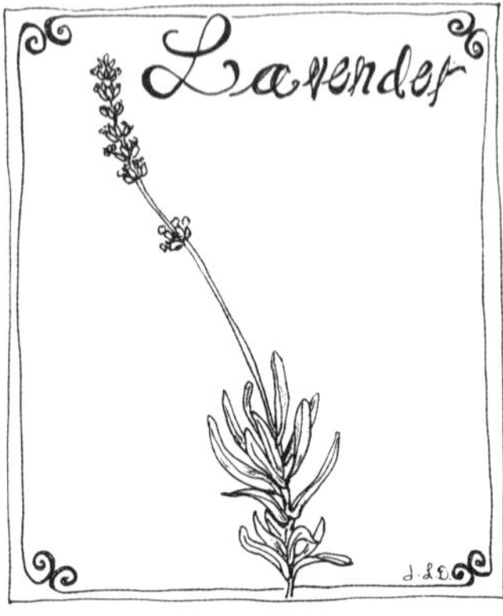

Lavender infused in oil makes a wonderful base for healing and soothing ointments. The oil itself also makes a very relaxing rub for sore, strained, overused muscles and painful joints.

· Lavender essential oil is excellent for treating minor burns and sunburn, helping to heal skin tissue and prevent scarring. Dilute with aloe vera gel and apply liberally and often!

· The above mixture may also be used to treat acne. Simply spread over face and allow to dry.

· To ease tired feet, combine 1 Tbsp. sea salt and ¼ cup dried lavender in a basin. Cover with boiling water and stir to blend; cool mixture until comfortable. Soak feet until water is cold.

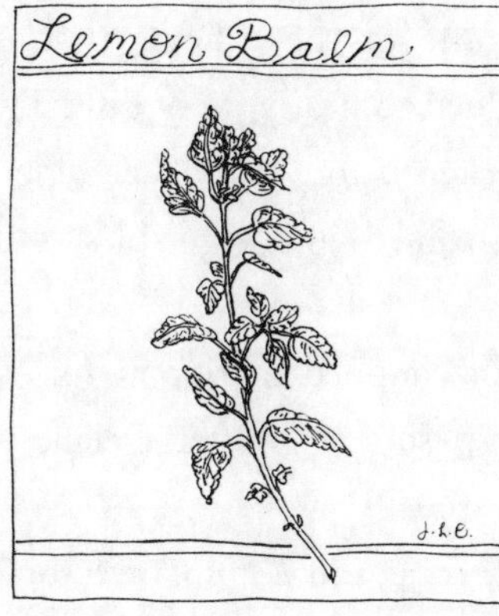

Lemon balm makes an extraordinarily relaxing tea when blended with chamomile and catnip.

· As a tea, lemon balm does more than relax the body: it is beneficial for maintaining digestive health, strengthening the immune system, and fighting winter illnesses.

· Need to ease nerves and relax tense muscles? Make a strong infusion of lemon balm and lavender in water. Strain out plant material and pour infusion into bath water. This also treats painful muscles and joints. And it cleanses, refreshes, and heals the skin too!

· Remember, lemon balm can slightly inhibit the thyroid-stimulating hormone. If you have thyroid problems, consult your health care provider before frequent use or high doses of this herb.

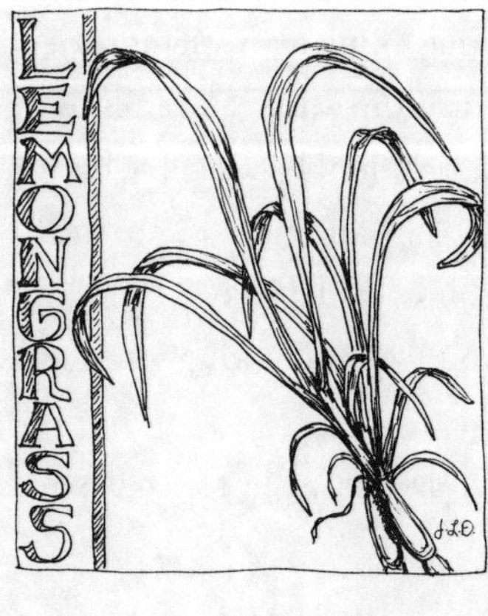

When baking a whole chicken, sprinkle lemon pepper seasoning over the top, then add fresh lemongrass leaves to the water in the bottom of the pan before baking. Discard leaves before serving. A truly tasty dish!

· Lemongrass is a wonderful addition to sleep pillows and bath sachets.

· The essential oil of lemongrass is quite strong, and powerful for treating skin problems. Add some to your favorite balm and apply to bruises for prompt healing.

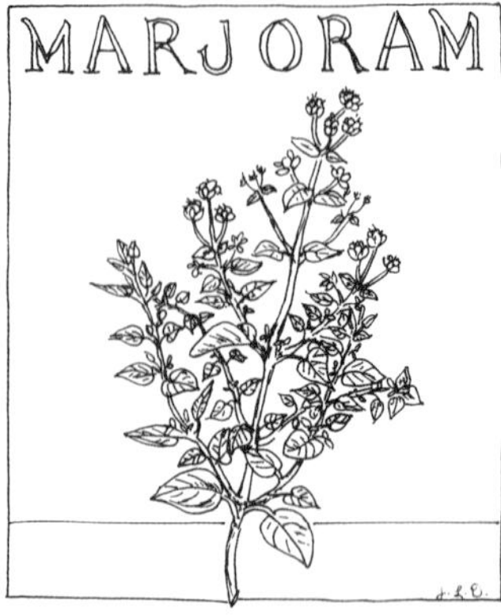

Marjoram is one of those herbs that is delicious added to nearly every dish! Try it sprinkled over chicken before you bake, added to poultry stuffing, steamed with vegetables, and the list goes on!

· Blend 1 Tbsp. fresh chopped marjoram (or ½ Tbsp. dry) with 8 Tbsp. softened butter. Delicious as a turkey sandwich spread!

· When making potato soup, add 2 Tbsp. fresh (or 2 tsp. dried) marjoram near the end of cooking. Simmer for about 3 minutes. Perfect flavor combination!

· Remember, marjoram makes a healthful tea that is especially good for fighting the common cold. It can lower fevers, has antioxidant properties, and relieves indigestion too. Plus it's excellent, when you add honey, for soothing overused vocal cords and laryngitis.

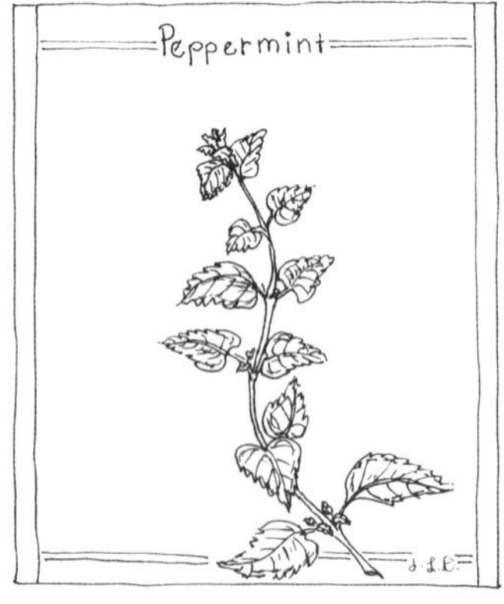

Add very strong mint tea to lemonade in place of part of the water. So refreshing!

· Place a few fresh or dried mint leaves in the bottom of a mug. Fill with hot chocolate for a tasty treat!

· To freshen breath and aid digestion, chew on a fresh mint leaf (as you would chewing gum) after a meal.

· The more you harvest mint, the faster it seems to grow!

· Adding a few mint leaves to baked pears or apples lends a pleasant flavor.

· Mint leaves are carefree garnishes, keeping their fresh, green beauty longer than most herbs.

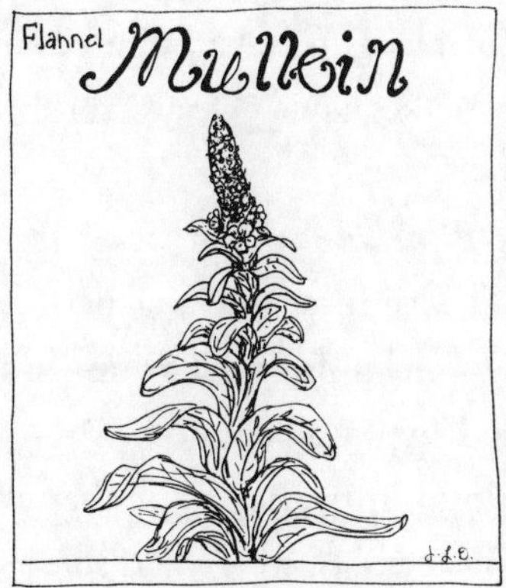

If you dislike the taste of mullein brewed in water, try brewing it in milk.

· You may use mullein infused oil as a warm oil treatment for dry, brittle hair. Warm the oil, massage into scalp and hair, cover with a plastic shower cap, and wrap with a towel that has been dipped into hot water and wrung out. Reheat the towel each time it cools. Leave on for 10 minutes or more. Gently shampoo.

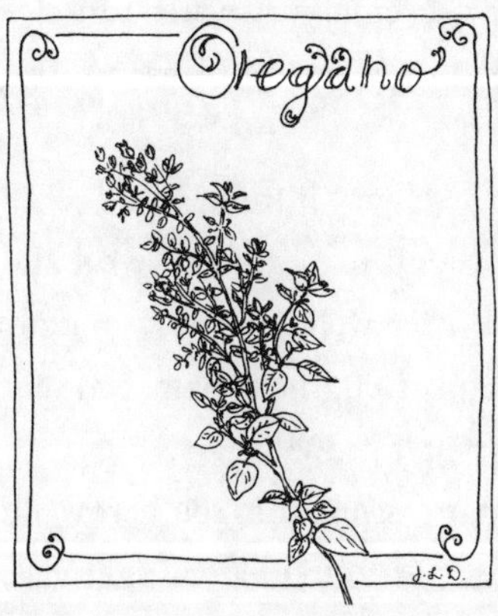

Oregano's appetizing flavor blends well with stews and casseroles.

· Try fresh oregano tossed with salad greens and topped with crumbled blue cheese.

· Melt butter and add dried oregano. Serve with artichokes. Wonderful!

· Oregano perks up bland bean dishes.

· Make a sachet of dried oregano and tie under the bath faucet. The herb's antiseptic, cleansing properties will make your skin fresh and clean!

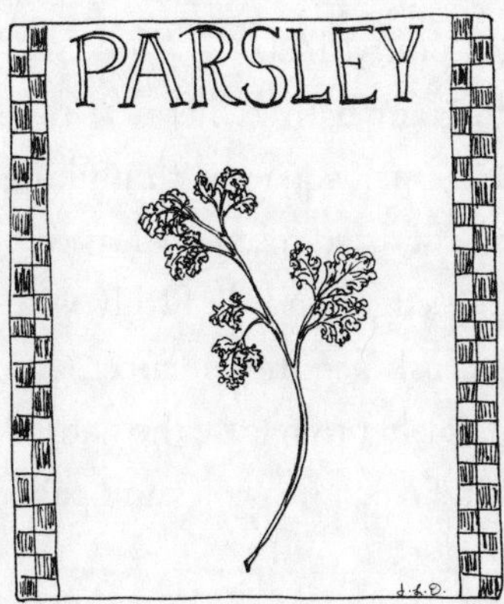

Add fresh chopped parsley and fresh snipped chives to your favorite succotash recipe. Yum!

· Remember, parsley sweetens the breath and soothes the digestive tract. Chew a sprig after a rich, spicy meal—especially one that's loaded with garlic!

· Parsley roots are a delicious treat—tender, crisp, and mild. Lightly steam, toss in butter, and enjoy! Or slice raw roots over salads.

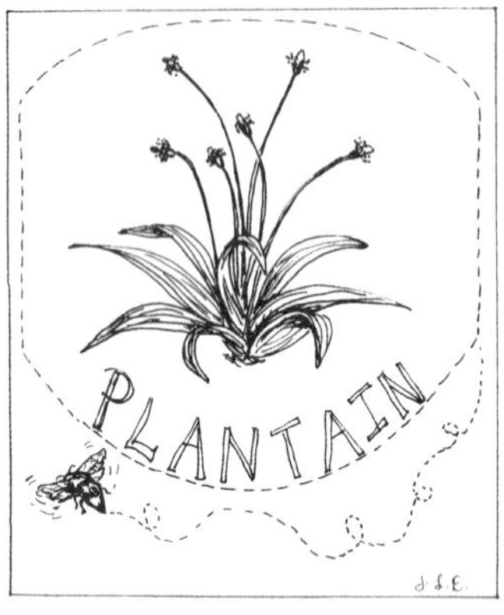

An infusion of plantain leaves, diluted in warm water, makes a deep-cleanse for the skin.

· Plantain (especially *P. media*) has a styptic effect on minor wounds. The infused oil is a perfect treatment for razor nicks from shaving—it's cleansing, healing, and styptic all at once!

· The above oil is helpful in treating a number of ailments, including blisters, bee stings, and sores.

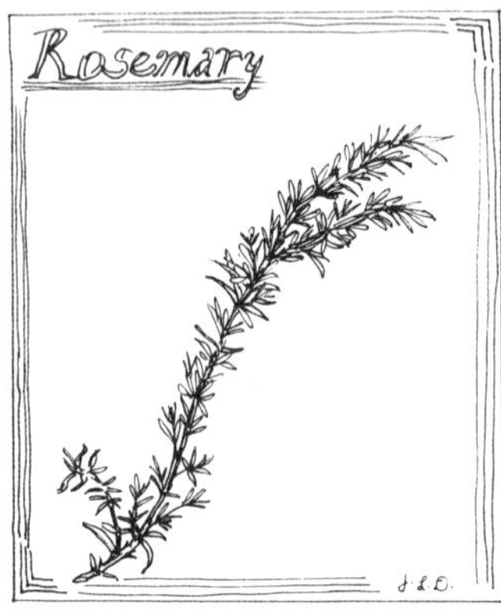

An infusion of rosemary in water can also be diluted and used as a hair rinse to treat dandruff.

· Add about 2 Tbsp. rosemary infused water to 12 ounces of shampoo. Blend in ½ tsp. olive oil and 1 Tbsp. aloe vera gel. Mix well and use as a daily shampoo that heals and strengthens damaged hair and promotes healthy hair growth.

· If you infuse rosemary, sage, and southernwood in olive oil, then strain and store in an airtight glass container, it makes a gentle hair restorative. Gently rub into scalp; let sit for 5 minutes; shampoo as usual.

· Add sprigs of rosemary to bouquets of cut flowers for extra fragrance and pretty filler.

· For a revitalizing, fragrant bath sachet, use thin cotton fabric cut into a small square with pinking shears; place a little pile of dried rosemary leaves in the middle. Gather the edges and tie firmly with twine. To use, gently crush bag, tie to faucet, and run hot water over the sachet to release the natural oils into the bath water. Soak away aches and pains and feel energized.

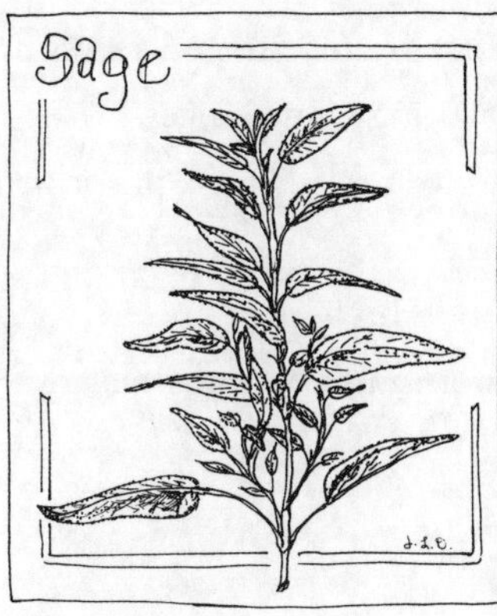

Sage blends deliciously well with sausage, while assisting the body in digestion!

· Add to pea soup, bean dishes, chowders, and stews.

· Chop 2 Tbsp. fresh sage and add to biscuit batter for a flavorful flair!

· Add to creamy cheddar cheese dips.

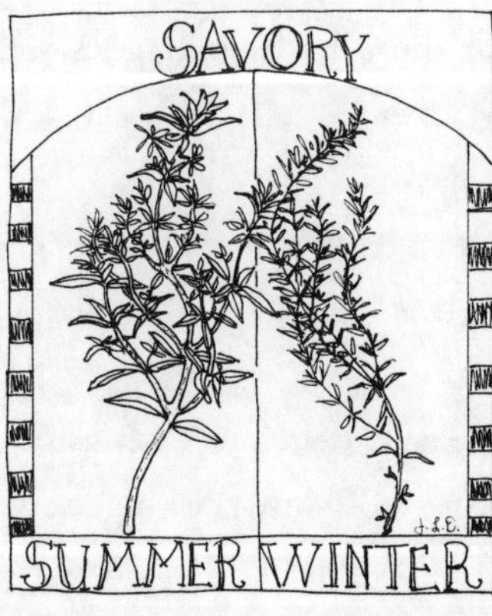

Add savory to slow-cooking soups and stews. Unlike some herbs, savory doesn't lose its flavor when cooked.

· Sprinkle a teaspoon of dried savory into gravies and white sauces.

· Dried savory makes a perky addition to bread crumbs for breading fish or chicken.

· Mix fresh savory with lemon juice, vinegar, minced garlic cloves, and honey for a flavorful marinade.

· Don't forget to add fresh savory leaves to your next garden salad—it's delicious!

· Use finely crushed savory as you would black pepper.

· Finely chop fresh savory and add to biscuit or dumpling batter.

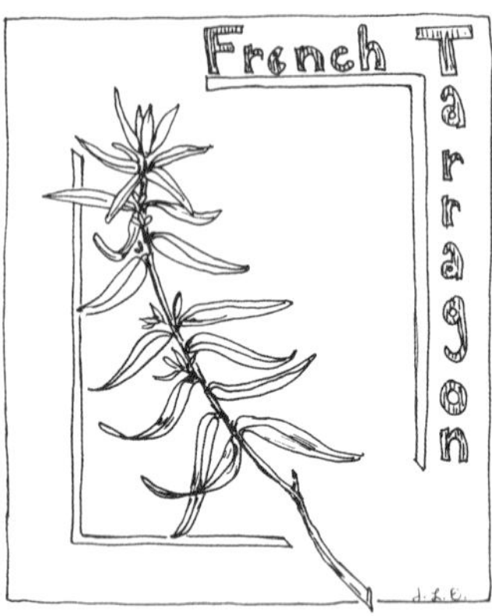

The hot, pungent taste of tarragon leaves are delicious for flavoring white sauces.

· Toss fresh leaves in green salads for a flavor perk and a nutritional boost!

· Tarragon makes wonderful herbed butter!

· Excellent flavoring for mustards and vinegar.

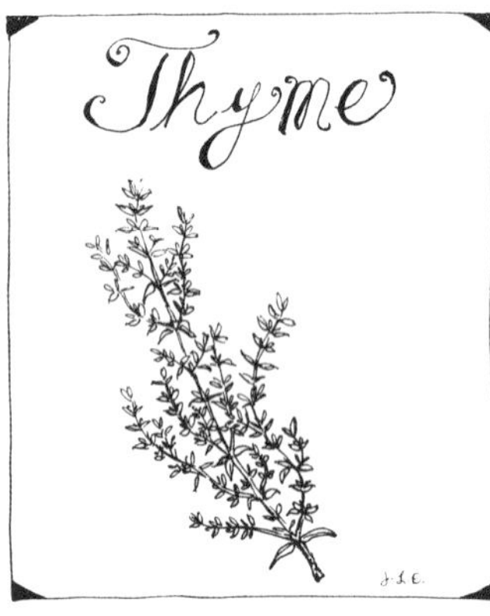

Thyme is one of those herbs that goes well with so many dishes—especially since it comes in a variety of flavors!

· Don't forget that lemon and lime thyme can be used for delicious teas, added to sorbet or ice cream, and so much more!

· Lemon thyme is especially delicious with fish.

· You can add thyme to slow-cooking stews or sauces (such as Italian sauces). The flavor is intensified by heat.

· Thyme is especially tasty with tomatoes.

USEFUL HINTS

Sprays of tansy scattered on the buffet table will help repel flies. (Don't eat the tansy—it's too bitter for consumption!)

· It increases the flavor to crush fresh leaves or crumble dried ones just before using.

· 1 Tbsp. of fresh herbs is usually equal to 1 tsp. of dried.

· It is best to harvest herbs in the coolness of a sunny morning, just as the dew has dried on the leaves.

· Harvest leaves just before the flowers bloom—that is when the herb's oil and/or flavor is at its peak.

· Freshly harvested herbs are usually the *best* for flavor. You can keep fresh-cut herbs fresh for about a week if you place a bouquet of them in a jar of water in the refrigerator and loosely cover the tops with a plastic bag.

· Not all herbs do well when dried in the microwave, but mint is an exception. Just lay a double layer of microwave-safe paper towels in your microwave, spread with fresh mint (only the soft stems and leaves), and microwave on high for about 3-4 minutes (when the leaves crumble between your fingers).

· A small mortar (sturdy bowl-shaped vessel) and pestle (club-shaped utensil) are an inexpensive investment you'll find indispensable for cooking with herbs—especially to crush dried seeds.

· A mortar and pestle are also useful for perking up dried herbs. Crush gently with pestle to release flavor before adding herbs to your cooking.

· Store dried herbs in airtight containers, in a place away from sunlight and heat. A cool, dark cupboard is the ideal location.

· Freeze blossoms of edible flowers in ice cubes. Serve with lemonade for a cheerful touch to any summertime event!

· *Bouquet garni* is the French term for several herbs tied in a piece of cheesecloth and added to slow-cooking dishes (such as stews). Add your favorite blend, or try the traditional thyme, parsley, and bay leaf blend.

Heartwarming Herbal Gifts

Blessed be the Lord, who daily loadeth us with benefits (Psalm 68:19).

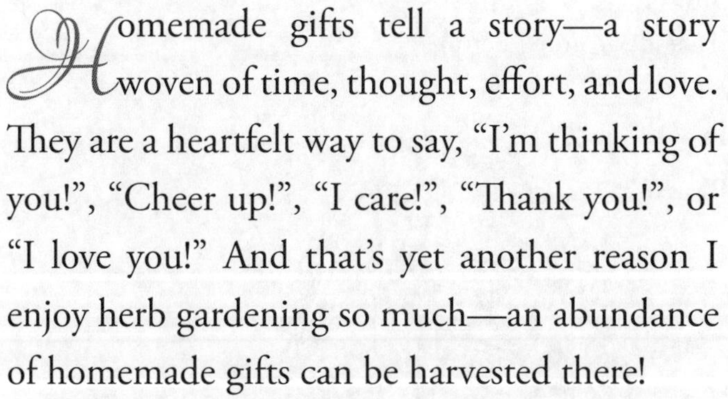

Homemade gifts tell a story—a story woven of time, thought, effort, and love. They are a heartfelt way to say, "I'm thinking of you!", "Cheer up!", "I care!", "Thank you!", or "I love you!" And that's yet another reason I enjoy herb gardening so much—an abundance of homemade gifts can be harvested there!

The following pages are crammed full of ideas. And that is just to get you started. I know it will spark your imagination and soon you'll be creating gifts you've dreamed up on your own! But for now, brew a cup of tea, find a comfortable chair, put up your feet, and enjoy the next few pages!

It is more blessed to give than to receive (Acts 20:35).

GIFT BASKETS

One of my favorite homemade gift projects is gift baskets. It's so easy to center them around the occasion, the receiver's interests, and so on. The following ideas are simple, fun, and well received!

TIME-FOR-YOU LAVENDER GIFT BASKET

Choose any shape or size basket you like!

Lavender-colored or print fabric
Matching thread and purple embroidery floss
1 cup dried lavender parts
Odds and ends of lavender-colored crayons (equaling about 1 cup)
1 tablespoon dried lavender
6 drops lavender oil
About ¼ yard of lavender-colored netting
3 yd. purple ribbon
3 yd. white ribbon
Candle wick (two 3" pieces)

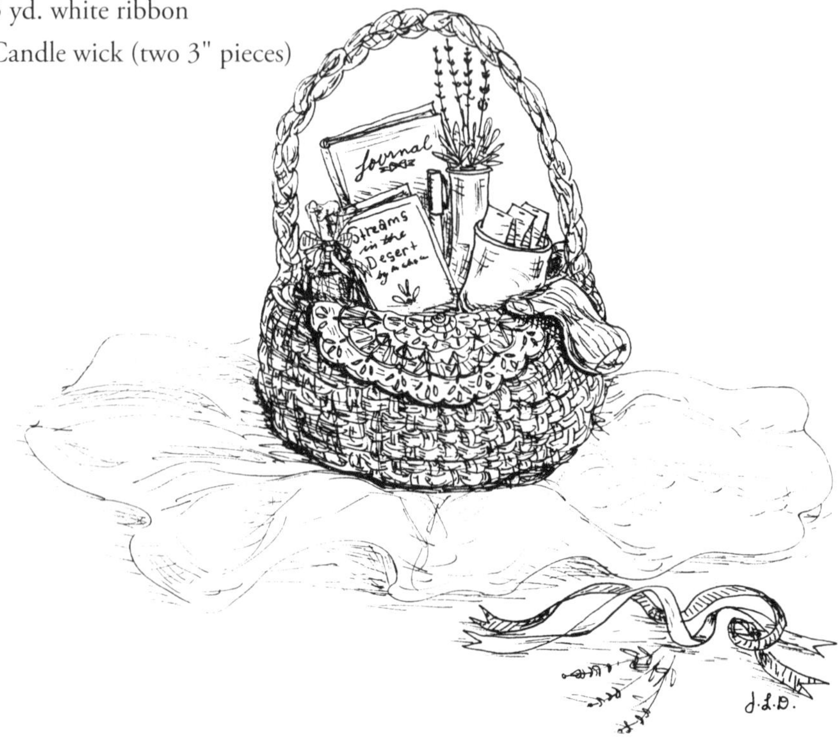

A devotional book

A lavender-colored journal and pen with purple ink

Mint tea bags

A teacup in lavender colors

A spray of dried lavender stalks with flowers, placed in a small glass vase

A white crocheted doily

Cozy white- or lavender-colored slipper socks

On a piece of paper, roughly trace the inside circumference of the basket. Trim paper with scissors until it fits comfortably into the bottom of the basket. Remove the paper and lay over doubled fabric (right sides together). Trace about ¼" larger than the paper is. Cut out fabric and sew all around the circle, leaving a 2" opening. Turn right-side-out and fill with 1 cup dried lavender. Whipstitch the opening. Gently crush and distribute the lavender inside the fabric circle. (Mmmmm—it smells *so-o-o* good!) Quilt with embroidery floss. Place in bottom of basket.

For the candles, in a double boiler (used for such purposes), place the crayon bits in the top. Fill the bottom with water. Gently melt the crayons; blend in dried lavender and essential oil. Pour into 2 greased molds, inserting candle wick in each candle. Remove candles when firm and wrap in squares of lavender-colored netting, tying with about 12" lengths of both ribbons. Place in basket.

Tie mint tea bags in a stack with about 24" of both ribbons; tuck into the teacup and place in the basket. Arrange remaining gifts in the basket. Center basket on a large square of lavender-colored netting; gather up the edges and tie with remaining ribbon. Tuck a spray of dried lavender into the bow. Add a homemade card. The perfect gift!

A homemade gift is a heartfelt way
to say, "Thank you!" or "I love you!"

MORE GIFT BASKET IDEAS!

The Herb Gardener's Basket—This is a fun basket to fill! Tuck in seed packets (perhaps seeds gathered from your own garden), homemade herbal hand salve, a refreshing and rejuvenating rosemary bath sachet, a bar of homemade herbal soap, a spray bottle of homemade herbal insect repellent, gardening gloves, and a small potted herb (such as lemon thyme).

Beat-the-Sniffles Basket—Here's a thoughtful gift for someone who is suffering from a bad cold! A small jar of honey and a spoon; a teacup with a cheery pattern; home-filled tea bags of chamomile, mint, and echinacea blend; a small airtight jar of horehound candy; a healing salve of lavender, comfrey, mint, and vitamin E (to soothe the outside of that sore, battered nose!); a good, uplifting book; and a small box of facial tissues.

Wildflower Herb Basket—This is a bright, cheery summer basket! Use flower-printed fabric and follow the instructions for filling the "Time-for-You Lavender Gift Basket" liner. Fill with dried herbs of your choice. Place in a basket. Tuck in calendula, sunflower, echinacea, and borage seed packets. Snuggle in a potted echinacea (in bloom!) from your own garden. Add handheld garden tools such as a trowel and cultivator. Arrange next to a small box of all-purpose Miracle-Gro™ and gardening gloves. You can also add a book on herb gardening and maybe a pretty hand-painted plaque with a garden theme.

"For You, Mom!" Basket—What are some of your mom's favorite things in life? Cooking? Reading? Writing? Gardening? Let her know you care about her by centering your theme around what she enjoys, and incorporating her favorite herbs into sachets, scented candles, herbal lotion, lip balm, foot soak mixes, and more!

Faithful Friends Basket—Friends are a gift from God. Take time to let your friends know they're special by putting together a basket with a friendship theme! Rosemary means "remembrance," so twine some stalks around the basket handle. Include things your friend loves best—a book with a homemade bookmark (using pressed herbs as embellishments), some of her favorite herbal tea and a teacup, a homemade friendship-themed plaque, a packet of note cards, and a pretty pen.

Baskets for dads, brothers, etc.—These are fun to make! Follow the instructions in "Time-for-You Lavender Gift Basket" for lining the basket. Use fabric with manly themes, such as nature, fishing, etc. Fill with shredded paper (for filler) and bay leaves (for fragrance). Add a book you know they'd enjoy, a homemade (dried-herb-embellished) bookmark, and a relaxing mint foot soak mix. Tuck in packets of hot chocolate and mint tea bags (the combination is delicious!) and a large mug.

Any blessing which we enjoy…is the gift of Him who is the great Author of good and the Father of mercies. –Joseph Addison

PRESSED HERBS

Many herbs make lovely pressed flowers and foliage—which opens up a huge assortment of gifts to make! Select herbs such as clover, yarrow, lavender, lobelia, mullein, catnip, echinacea, or roses. If you have a flower press, wonderful! If not, gather a stack of large, heavy books. I like to use an old phone book to actually place the herbs in, which prevents messing up the pages of other books. Open the old phone book in the center, lay a piece of blotting paper on one side, and arrange plant material. Place squares of blotting paper over the thinner parts so that everything will press evenly. Cover with another piece of blotting paper and carefully close phone book. Lay on top of a hardcover book, place another hardcover book on top of the phone book and secure all together with thick rubber bands. Stack heavy books on top. The next day, carefully check your herbs. Is the blotting paper wet? Replace the paper carefully (tweezers help!) and put everything back in place. Leave in the "press" for about six weeks. (Check every few days—but be careful not to disturb things too much!) When they are completely dry you may begin your gift projects!

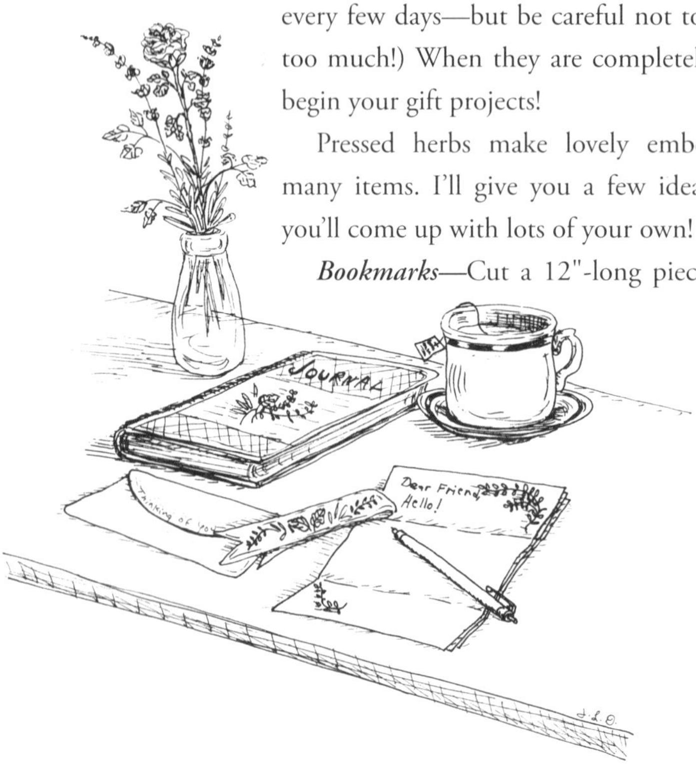

Pressed herbs make lovely embellishments for many items. I'll give you a few ideas, and I know you'll come up with lots of your own!

Bookmarks—Cut a 12"-long piece of wide satin ribbon; bend in half lengthwise and cut bottom into an inverted "V". Drizzle a thin pattern of puzzle glue along the front 6" of your bookmark. Carefully arrange plant material and hang to dry. Very gently brush a layer of puzzle glue over the dried herbs and hang to dry again. When clear and dry, tuck into a book as a thoughtful gift! You may also follow the instructions for journal covers (below), using a strip of cardboard for a bookmark base in place of a ribbon.

Homemade cards, stationery, and journal covers—Arrange your choice of dried herbs. Using small drops of school glue, carefully glue in place. For journal covers, allow glue to dry completely and cover the whole area with contact paper.

Decorated gift soap—Moisten the top of a bar of soap. Melt a small amount of beeswax and brush on the underside of the dried flowers or leaves. Gently press in place. Allow to dry completely. Seal in plastic wrap.

Easy Glycerin Soap

3 (16 oz.) blocks pure glycerin, divided
(available through Lehman's Non-electric; see page 224)
6 drops essential oil of your choice, divided
12 pressed herb leaves
12 pressed herb flowers
non-stick cooking spray

Coat a 12-cup muffin pan with non-stick cooking spray. In the top of a double boiler, melt 1½ blocks glycerin. Stir in 3 drops essential oil; fill muffin cups half full with mixture. Let firm. Arrange dried botanicals over firmed mixture. Melt remaining glycerin and add remaining essential oil. Top off muffin cups. Let cook completely; invert on waxed paper. When completely cool and firm, wrap individual bars in plastic wrap.

Take time today to let your loved ones know you care—
there may not be a tomorrow!

OTHER FUN HERBAL GIFTS

- Fill your own tea bags, label, and arrange in a pretty teacup or manly mug.
- Dried herbs can be woven into a grapevine wreath for a homey, fragrant wall hanging. A lovely gift!
- Do you make your own herbal soaps, salves, creams, or ointments? These make delightful (and much-appreciated!) gifts.
- Sachets are simple and sweet gifts. With a variety of dried herbs and cotton fabric scraps, you can make relaxing bath sachets, revitalizing foot-soak sachets, fragrant moth-repelling linen sachets, room-freshener sachets, and so much more! Label each one and include instructions.
- Potpourri makes a nice gift too! Mix together fragrant herbs and spices, sprinkle in a few drops of essential oil, and place in a pretty potpourri container.
- *Bouquet garni,* seasoning herbs tucked into cheesecloth and tied with kitchen string, make a perfect gift for the cook. Place the bundles in a shiny new kettle with a pretty cotton bag of dried beans and a bean soup recipe.
- Keep your eyes open for small wooden coat racks (the kind you hang on a wall) at yard sales and thrift stores. Sand the rack and paint it a nice color. Pick bouquets of herbs in bloom (such as roses, lavender, and rosemary). Tie each bouquet with matching ribbon and hang upside-down from the pegs on the coat rack. When the herbs are completely dry, it's ready to give away. Now that's a pretty gift!
- So many herbal gift arrangements go well with teacups or mugs. I like to keep my eyes open for bargains at yard sales and thrift stores—you find such unique, lovely cups for next to nothing! Last summer I discovered a cute white teacup with an old-fashioned picture on it of a mother reading her child a bedtime story. It reminded me of my childhood! And therefore made the perfect gift—with some lemony herb tea tucked in—for my mother. By the way, it was only $2!

· Certain perennial herbs benefit from being divided in the fall or spring. If your bushes are getting overgrown, divide them and place some in pots. Keep them well cared for until they are established, and then give the lovely potted herbs to your friends!

· Next time you make rye bread, bursting with caraway seeds, double the batch and give a loaf to a friend. If you want to make the gift extra special, wrap the loaf in plastic wrap and place it in a large bread basket with a plate (purchased at a yard sale or thrift store), a jar of homemade herbal cheese spread, a butter knife, and a pretty tea towel.

· Do you have a "secret" pickle recipe everybody asks for? If you don't want to give out the recipe, simply give jars of your special pickles! Or if you want to share, write the recipe out on a recipe card and use rickrack to tie it around the lid of the jar.

Homemade herbal gifts… I think you'll agree that they're unique, lovely, and special! Why not write a list of your own ideas and get started? It's an adventure for your creativity, and a wonderful way to share the bounty of your herb garden. Have fun—and know that those who receive your gifts will too!

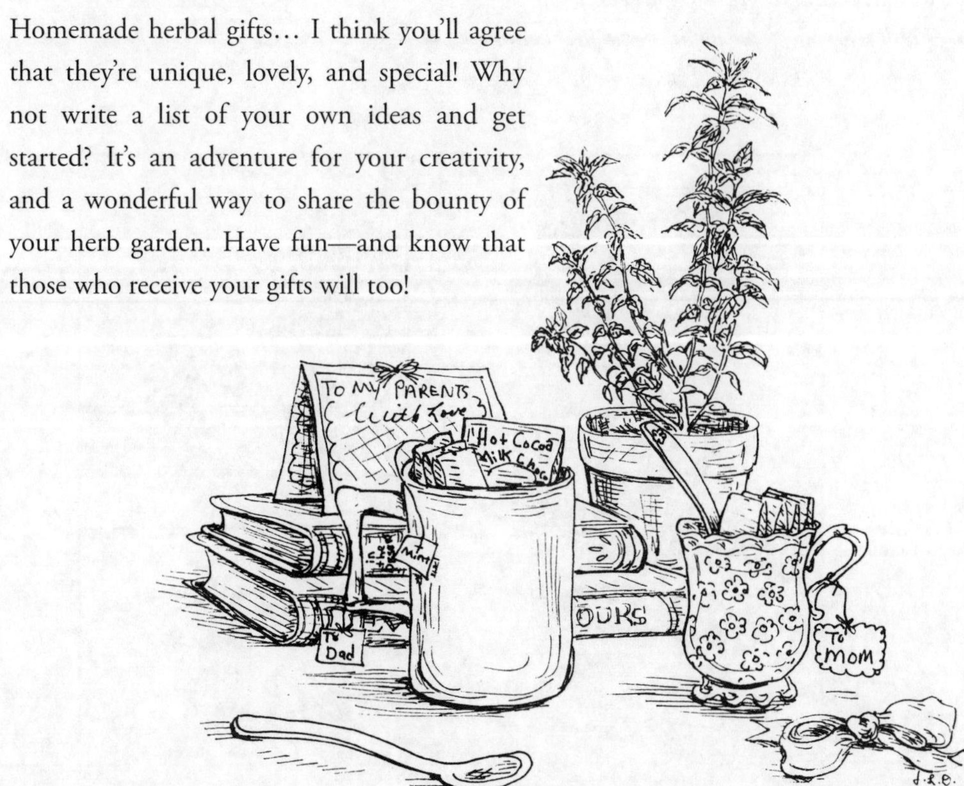

A Simple Sachet

It was just a small calico square
(And yet tucked inside, wafting scent most fair,
Was a gift that came from the work of years),
With the edges trimmed by
some pinking shears.

Yes, the gift she gave is a special one—
So I smile my thanks for the work she's done.
It's a homemade gift (with a history)
That she took the time to make just for me!

Do you wonder why I enjoy it so—
Such a simple gift without cost or show?
I will tell you, then, what the sachet means—
How it speaks to me of sweet, homey things!

The rose petals came from her mother. She
Brought the rosebush from the old country.
And the lavender? From a fine old plant
She was given once by her favorite aunt.

And the bay leaves came from the potted tree
That they've kept for years on their balcony.
And the ribbon tied in a bow on top?
Well, she found it once in a fabric shop.

–J.L.D.

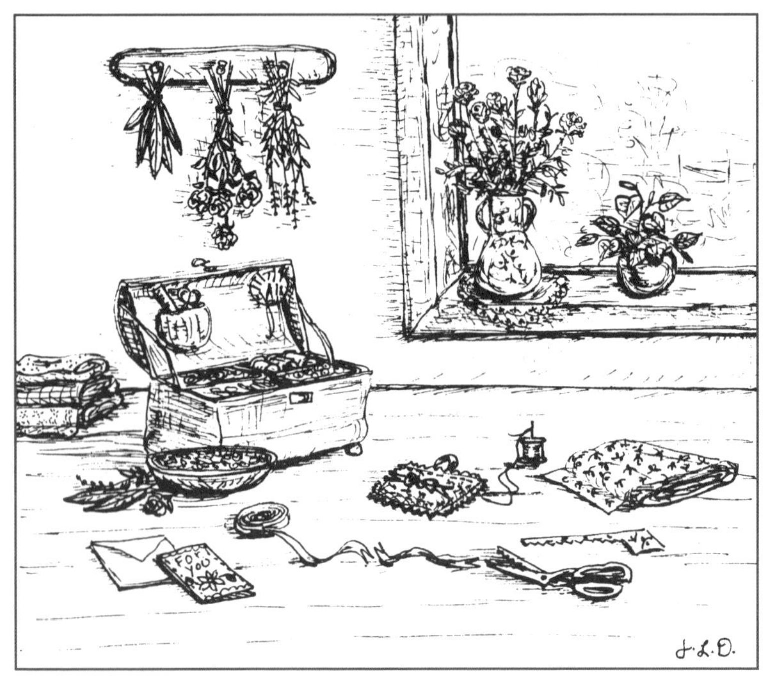

Resources

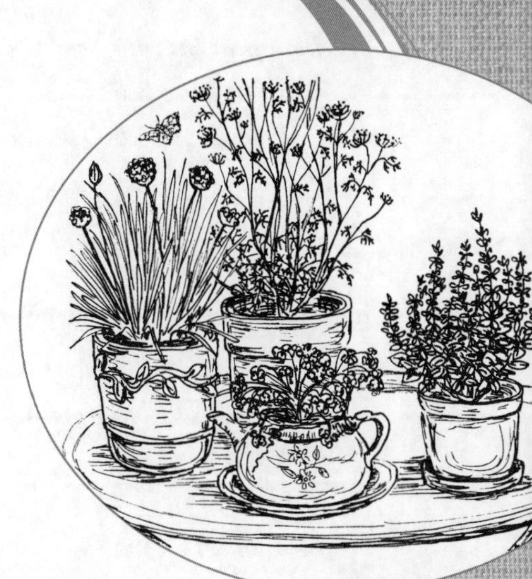

Backyard Herbs and Flowers
8128 Maurer Road
Apple Creek, OH 44606

A beautiful, informative catalog! This family-operated company offers plants, garlic, seeds, books, tincture kits, bulk dried herbs and herbal tea blends, iron-close fill-your-own tea bags, glass tincture bottles, salve containers, and so much more! Reasonable prices. Highly recommended!

Berlin Seeds
5335 County Road 77
Millersburg, OH 44654
Phone: 1-877-464-0892

Full-color catalog brimming with seeds, plants, fertilizers, pest/disease controls, tools, cookware, books, accessories—and much more! This is one of my favorite catalog companies! Highly recommended.

Botanical Interests Seed Catolog
660 Compton Street
Broomfield, CO 80020
Phone: 1-800-821-4340

Full-color catalog with a wonderful selection of herb, vegetable, and flower seeds! Lime basil seeds are sold here. Each packet includes how-tos and recipes! Informative articles. Excellent catalog.

Lehman's Non-Electric Catalog
One Lehman Circle
PO Box 41
Kidron, OH 44636
Phone: 1-877-438-5346

If you don't already get this catalog, send for it today! It's packed with wonderful products—including that oh-so-useful potato ricer and French press coffeemaker. They also carry reusable cheesecloth and other products helpful in making herbal preparations, such as stainless steel funnels and double boilers. Keep your eyes open for gardening tools, a plethora of soap making supplies (including pure glycerin blocks that are perfect for melting down and adding essential oils, infused oils, etc.!), and so much more!

Bulk Herb Store
26 West 6th Ave.
Lobelville, TN 37097
Phone: 1-877-278-4257

Many quality herbs, books, and products. Vegetable glycerin, tea infusers, press-and-brew tea bags, tea mixes, tincture kits, and more.

Walnut Creek Botanicals
2325 TR 444
Sugarcreek, OH 44681
Phone: 330-893-1095

Their herbal tincture kits make it easy for anyone to get started making their own herbal remedies.

Gardens Alive!
5100 Schenley Place
Lawrenceburg, IN 47025
Phone: 513-354-1482

Organic pest and insect controls, fertilizers, etc. This full-color catalog is as useful as a book, including a large guide to insect pests and diseases, and how to control them naturally.

Nature's Warehouse
PO Box 682
Theresa, NY 13691
Phone: 1-800-215-4372

Large, full-color catalog filled with quality products—vitamins, minerals, bulk herbs, essential oils, body care products, books, accessories, and *much* more. Amber glass dropper bottles available here! This quarterly catalog also contains insightful articles on healthy living. Highly recommended.

Herbal Recipes for Vibrant Health, by Rosemary Gladstar. Helpful for learning herbal preparations and dosage. May be purchased through *Backyard Herbs and Flowers* catalog.

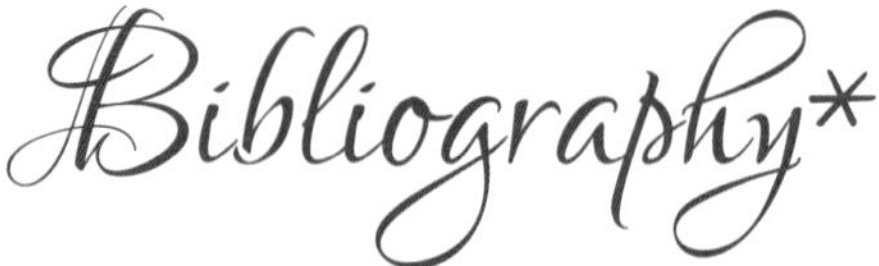

Balch, CNC Phyllis A. and James F. Balch, MD. *Prescription for Nutritional Healing*, 3rd Edition. New York: Avery: A Member of Penguin Putnam, Inc., 375 Hudson Street, New York, NY 10014. 2000.

Bremness, Lesley. *The Complete Book of Herbs: A Practical Guide to Growing and Using Herbs*. New York: Penguin Studio, The Penguin Group. 375 Hudson Street, New York, NY 10014. 1988.

Cutler, Karen Davis. *A Burpee Book: The Complete Vegetable and Herb Gardener*. New York: Macmillan, A Simon and Schuster Macmillan Company, 1633 Broadway, New York, NY 10019. 1997.

The Editors of Storey Books. *Country Wisdom and Know-How*. New York: Storey Publishing LLC, Black Dog and Leventhal Publishers, Inc., 151 West 19th Street, New York, NY 10011. 2004.

Emery, Carla. *The Encyclopedia of Country Living, Updated Ninth Edition*. Washington: Sasquatch Books, 119 South Main Street, Suite 400, Seattle, WA 98104. 2003.

Garland, Sarah. *The Complete Book of Herbs and Spices*. New York: A Reader's Digest Book, The Reader's Digest Association, Inc., Pleasantville, New York. 1983.

Hartung, MH Tammi. *Growing 101 Herbs that Heal*. Vermont: Storey Books, Pownal, VT 05261. 2000.

Hemphill, John and Rosemary, *What Herb Is That?* Pennsylvania: Stackpole Books, 5067 Ritter Road, Mechanicsburg, PA 17055. 1995.

Keville, Kathi. *Herbs: An Illustrated Encyclopedia*. New York: Friedman/Fairfax Publishers, 15 West 26 Street, New York, NY 10010. 1994.

**Note: Most of these books contain subtle New Age beliefs that the author does not endorse or agree with.*

Hardiness Zone Map

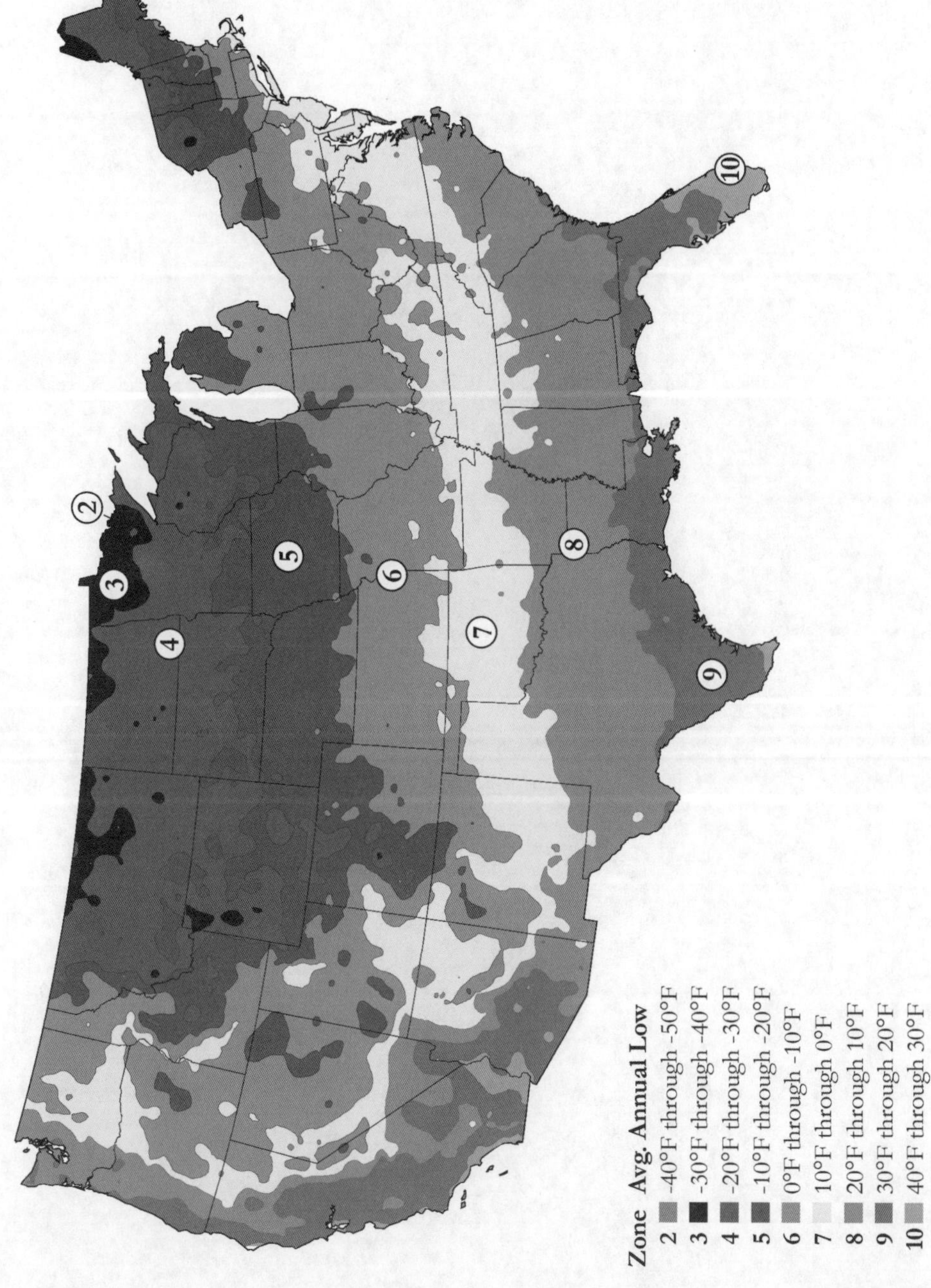

Index

R

S

T

V

W